# Principles of
# Neurologic Diagnosis

**Little, Brown
and Company
Boston/Toronto**

# Principles of Neurologic Diagnosis

## Erwin B. Montgomery, Jr., M.D.
*Assistant Professor of Neurology, Department of Neurology and Neurosurgery, Washington University School of Medicine, St. Louis, Missouri; Attending Physician, Department of Neurology, Barnes Hospital, St. Louis*

## Michael Wall, M.D.
*Associate Professor of Neurology and Ophthalmology, Tulane University School of Medicine, New Orleans, Louisiana; Attending Physician, Tulane Medical Center and The Charity Hospital at New Orleans*

## Victor W. Henderson, M.D.
*Associate Professor of Neurology and Gerontology, University of Southern California School of Medicine, and the Ethel Percy Andrus Gerontology Center, Los Angeles, California; Co-Director, University of Southern California Neurobehavior Clinic/ Bowles Center for Alzheimer's and Related Diseases, Los Angeles*

Copyright © 1986 by Erwin D. Montgomery, Jr., M.D., Michael Wall, M.D., and Victor W. Henderson, M.D.

First Edition

*Third Printing*

All rights reserved. No part of this book may be reproduced in any form or by any electronic or mechanical means, including information storage and retrieval systems, without permission in writing from the publisher, except by a reviewer who may quote brief passages in a review.

Library of Congress Catalog Card No. 85-080755

ISBN 0-316-57867-3

Printed in the United States of America

RRD VA

To our tolerant and enduring families

**Contents**

Preface xi
Acknowledgments xiii
Introduction 3

Case 1. Weakness of the Right Arm and Leg and Numbness of the Left Arm and Leg 11

Case 2. Right-Sided Weakness and Left Gaze Paresis 23

Case 3. Right-Sided Weakness and Double Vision 37

Case 4. Weakness of Both Lower Extremities 47

Case 5. Dizziness, Ataxia, Right Arm Clumsiness, and Right-Sided Decreased Sensation 59

Case 6. Loss of Vision in the Right Eye, History of Right-Sided Weakness and Left-Sided Numbness 69

Case 7. Left-Sided Weakness, Left Gaze Paresis, and Left Visual Field Loss 79

Case 8. Galactorrhea and Double Vision 91

Case 9. Visual Loss with Olfactory Hallucinations and Altered Behavior 99

Case 10. Sudden Difficulty Speaking 107

Case 11. Left-Sided Weakness and Perceptual Disturbances 117

Case 12. Right Visual Field Loss and Alexia 125

Case 13. Speech Difficulty, Right-Sided Weakness, and Clumsiness of the Left Hand 135

Case 14. Gait and Truncal Ataxia and Headache 151

Case 15. Ataxia and Weakness of the Left Arm 159

Case 16. Unconsciousness, Left-Sided Weakness, and Dysconjugate Gaze  169
Case 17. Unconsciousness, Altered Respirations, and Left-Sided Weakness  183
Case 18. Unconsciousness  197
Case 19. Unresponsiveness and Ophthalmoplegia  203
Case 20. Weakness and Sensory Loss in the Right Hand  215
Case 21. Traumatic Weakness and Numbness of the Right Arm, with Anisocoria  227
Case 22. Double Vision and Facial Numbness  243
Case 23. Facial Weakness  251
Case 24. Difficulty Walking and Urinary Bladder Dysfunction  259

Index  271

# Preface

The bewilderment on the faces of some medical students and house officers confronting a problem in neurologic diagnosis stands in sharp contrast to our belief that neurology is, for the most part, quite straightforward. We wanted to develop a method of teaching an introduction to neurologic diagnosis that would emphasize a logical approach relying on anatomic and physiologic principles without requiring a prior knowledge of clinical neurology, thus ensuring feasibility and preventing frustration. Also, such an approach could be applied to almost any circumstance in neurology, whereas pattern recognition would be limited, particularly for the beginning student.

In writing this book and in discussions with friends and colleagues it became apparent that such an approach could not be derived from consideration of patient history and physical examination alone. Rather, this logical approach requires the development of a way of thinking, which then is applied to the patient history and physical examination and gives them context and relevance. Whereas many books on this subject have emphasized the history and physical examination, we have focused on the development of a way of thinking in anatomic and physiologic terms. In the cases presented in this book, the history and physical examinations are constructed (artificially at times) to emphasize the logical thinking processes involved. Our approach may not be the one used by experienced neurologists, but it does provide a framework for the fledgling neurologist to begin to understand clinical neurology.

E. B. M.
M. W.
V. W. H.

**Acknowledgments**

We thank Mr. Joseph S. Hayes for the illustrations, Ms. Patti Nacci for manuscript preparation, and Drs. William M. Landau and Joseph Green for their valuable comments.

E. B. M.
M. W.
V. W. H.

# Principles of
# Neurologic Diagnosis

# Introduction

# Introduction

Regardless of professional background, the newcomer can find neurologic diagnosis bewildering. Each patient presents an amalgamation of symptoms and signs, confusing because of the inherent complexity of the nervous system. A doctor unaccustomed to the process of neurologic diagnosis may fail to refer appropriate patients to a neurologist or refer needlessly. He may inappropriately perform laboratory procedures such as computerized tomographic (CT) scan, possibly causing unnecessary expense and, more dangerous, a false sense of security after a normal study. The impact of such errors is considerable, since neurologic diseases and neurologic complications of other diseases make up a significant portion of a general medical practice.

How does one make a neurologic diagnosis, and how does one teach others to do it? In general, there are several approaches.

The first approach is pattern recognition, whereby a neurologic diagnosis, such as a stroke or brain tumor, is intuitively inferred from a specific constellation of symptoms and signs. This approach has distinct drawbacks. It requires the accurate recall of many specific details relating to numerous disease entities and puts one at a significant disadvantage in dealing with an unusual disease or unusual manifestations of a common disease. To learn this approach, the only recourse is rote memorization, which most students find very unpleasant. Another disadvantage is that this approach does not suggest specific methods for eliciting the history, performing the physical examination, or delineating subsequent laboratory evaluation of the patient. It depends on the history and physical examination to produce symptoms and signs sufficient for pattern recognition. The only way to be sure that enough information has been obtained is to conduct a comprehensive examination. But what is sufficiently comprehensive?

A second approach is hypothesis testing. From the patient's initial complaints a diagnostic hypothesis is generated—for example, a stroke from occlusion of the middle cerebral artery. This hypothesis is then tested against data obtained from the history, physical examination, and laboratory evaluation. This approach has a major advantage in that the initial hypothesis need not be correct, since it may be revised as new data accumulate. Further, a particular method of examination is suggested, because only those issues relevant to the hypothesis need to be tested. This approach is not tied to any specific hypothesis and is well suited to the unusual situation.

However, the formulation of this approach overlooks the question "Where do the hypotheses to be tested come from?" The usual response is to fall back on pattern recognition, with its inherent limitations, described above. The hypothesis-testing approach may become an extension of the pattern recognition approach. With either, the student is condemned to memorization and repeated practice until neurology "makes sense"—that is, until the student recognizes enough patterns to begin to feel comfortable. This is how most neurologists learn and use neurology, and this is how most neurologists teach it.

There is a third approach, in which the initial effort is not to establish a neurologic diagnosis or hypothesis. Rather, the neurologic diagnosis follows from a logical chain of events (Fig. I-1) beginning with the development of an anatomic diagnosis (the identification of the anatomic site of the lesion) from an analysis of the patient's symptoms and signs. Once the anatomic diagnosis is made, the pathologic differential easily follows, since only certain types of

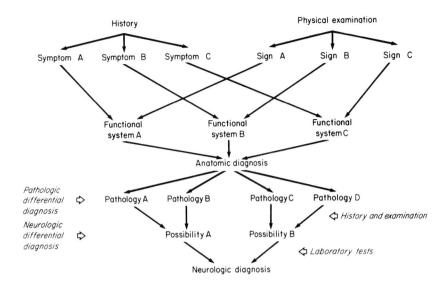

Figure I-1.

pathology are likely to occur at that anatomic site. From further consideration of the history and physical examination one selects likely pathologic possibilities for the neurologic differential diagnosis, which is further refined by the application of relevant laboratory testing.

This approach does not require the prior generation of a hypothesis of the neurologic diagnosis, as in the hypothesis-testing approach, and the diagnosis is deduced, not inferred as in the pattern recognition approach. The advantage of this third approach is that it requires only the basic knowledge, already possessed by most students, that is necessary to organize the patient's symptoms and signs into the major anatomic systems involved. Moreover, this approach does not preclude hypothesis testing or pattern recognition. Indeed, as the student gains more experience, he or she may increasingly use these methods. For the beginning student, however, the anatomic approach facilitates development of the skills of pattern recognition by demonstrating the anatomic and physiologic consistency of the patterns.

The anatomic approach is consistent with the fundamental importance of anatomy to the mechanisms of disease. The nervous system is limited in the way it reacts to injury. Usually there is a loss of function (e.g., blindness or weakness) or excess of function (e.g., seizures or tingling). In some cases complex functions of an otherwise intact area are altered by distant disconnecting lesions, which preclude input from other functional systems (the so-called disconnection syndromes). Therefore, the patient's symptoms and signs are more a result of *where* the nervous system is affected rather than of *what* is affecting the nervous system. An infarct of the motor cortex causes the same hemiplegia as does a tumor. It is true that symptoms of infarcts are usually sudden in onset while those of tumors are gradual, and this difference aids in the differential diagnosis; however, a significant percentage of tumors can present with sudden onset of symptoms and signs and can be confused with an infarct. The patient's symptoms and signs will most readily allow an anatomic localization of the lesion and, therefore, anatomic diagnosis rather than neurologic diagnosis.

In examining the patient, one can only observe the responses to various stimuli, ranging from complex questions and commands to the sudden stretch of a muscle tendon. Between the stimuli and the responses are numerous interactions at levels of the nervous system invisible to the examiner, which include the reception and interpretation of the stimuli; integration of the stimuli with the organism's current status and motivation; and formulation and performance of the response. Disorders of the nervous system can affect one or several of these levels. As a result, a given stimulus elicits different responses depending on what level of the nervous system is affected.

Neurology has been successful in recognizing how disorders at different levels of interaction influence the response to a given stimulus. For example, a patient who has a disturbance in the way he walks may be found to have a lesion (such as a tumor or infarct) of the cerebellum. When the same type of gait abnormality is observed in other patients, neurologists may infer that these patients also have cerebellar lesions. Thus, neurology has developed a functional anatomy of the nervous system. In this way lesions of various anatomic areas of the brain have been correlated with specific symptoms and signs. This knowledge is generalized so that when one examines a patient with certain abnormalities of function (i.e., symptoms and signs), one can deduce the specific anatomic area involved by the disease process.

A word of caution is in order. Although a system of functional anatomy has evolved in neurology, any classification is bound to be an oversimplification. Correlation of a function to a specific anatomic site can be considered only a general rule, for which there may be exceptions. Furthermore, abnormalities seen with nervous system disorders not only are the result of loss of function of the destroyed nervous structures but also reflect the attempts of the remaining structures to compensate. Therefore, the function of an area destroyed must be inferred indirectly from the abnormalities produced.

In the anatomic approach, when a patient presents with a variety of symptoms and signs, each symptom and sign is analyzed and a functional system involved by the disease process is identified. For example, weakness, spasticity, hyperreflexia, and Babinski's sign imply that the corticospinal system is involved. However, the corticospinal tract runs the entire length of the central nervous system, and further analysis is necessary to identify where the lesion is along the corticospinal system. These additional data come from a similar analysis of other related symptoms and signs, which identify other functional systems involved in the disease process. At this point the concept of parsimony, or Occam's razor, is employed (the fourteenth-century philosopher William of Occam said, "It is vain to do with more what can be done with fewer"). In neurologic terms, one tries to find the single anatomic site where a lesion can affect those functional systems identified as involved from the symptoms and signs and spare those systems thought to be intact. If one knows the anatomy of the functional systems involved, it is usually a relatively easy matter to identify the one anatomic site where the anatomic projections of the involved functional systems are in close proximity while those of the uninvolved systems are not. Thus the anatomic site of the disease process is identified, and this identification constitutes the anatomic diagnosis.

What about disorders of the nervous system refractory to discrete anatomic diagnosis of a single lesion? These disorders are few, but the concept of an anatomic diagnosis remains critical to their diagnosis. For example, the diagnosis of multiple sclerosis requires the presence of multiple lesions deduced from the history and physical examination. Therefore, the logical process of identifying the anatomic sites of several lesions is still necessary for the diagnosis of multiple sclerosis.

Future research will probably reduce further those disorders refractory to anatomic diagnosis and add new dimensions to the way anatomic diagnoses are achieved. Until recently the functional anatomy of the nervous system has been defined in terms of physiologic correlations with anatomy; for example, the nucleus cuneatus is correlated with sensations such as proprioception. More recent advances are now defining functional anatomy in terms of biochemical alterations, such as pathways utilizing specific neurotransmitters or metabolic functions; thus, Parkinson's disease may be considered a disorder of the dopaminergic neurotransmitter system. However, the concept of anatomic diagnosis remains critical to neurologic diagnoses.

Once the anatomic diagnosis has been made, the next step is to determine the cause. At each site there are a specific and limited number of types of pathology that can produce the anatomic lesion. There may be pathologic alterations of the tissue normally present: For example, meninges within or adjacent to the anatomic lesion may give rise to a meningioma; peripheral nerves, a neurofibroma; or glia, a glioma. In addition to pathologic alterations of tissues normally present, other disease processes tend to occur at a specific site: For example, sarcoidosis of the central nervous system (CNS) tends to affect the hypothalamus; tuberculosis affects the basal meninges. The list of possible types of pathology for a given nervous system locus is the pathologic differential diagnosis. Again, these hypotheses of the pathologic differential diagnosis are derived from the anatomic diagnosis, and not from recollection of long lists.

The pathologic differential diagnosis can be long and can include unlikely possibilities. The neurologic differential diagnosis represents the ordering of the pathologic possibilities according to probability, to exclude the unlikely possibilities. This is done by considering the patient's history and physical findings. From experience the neurologist knows that the sudden onset of symptoms implies disturbance in blood flow, migraine, trauma, or seizure. Thus, in the setting of a sudden onset of symptoms, those items in the pathologic differential diagnosis related to blood flow, migraine, trauma, or seizures are most probable. The gradual appearance of symptoms suggests an expanding lesion, such as a tumor. The patient's age also influences which items in the pathologic differential diagnosis are most likely; for example, childhood astrocytomas, unlike astrocytomas in adults, more often occur in the posterior fossa. The final step is to reduce the neurologic differential diagnosis to a single neurologic diagnosis. This may require laboratory tests ranging from computerized tomography to biopsy.

In this book, cases are presented to exemplify the processes as to how hypotheses are developed in clinical neurology. The facts of each case are given. At issue is what those facts mean to the physician, not how those facts were obtained. Thus, this book will largely ignore the mechanisms of history taking and physical examination. Some cases are "ideal" in that symptoms and signs not usually encountered are included to illustrate various principles. Some hypotheses (i.e., pathologic differential diagnoses) are considered for the sake of completeness rather than for their likelihood. Some of the logical processes may seem trivial for some of the cases, but they are used in a conscious and deliberate fashion to develop disciplined logic.

Just as in the development of any physical skill the beginner has to be consciously aware of the exact placement and movement of his extremities, so too the medical student may need to proceed in the same deliberate, stepwise fashion. With experience the processes will be internalized and implicitly used. With further experience, the clinician may be able immediately to recognize the disease in the patterns of symptoms and signs, just as the skilled craftsman seems to move almost reflexly. But such is not the situation in the beginning, and it is our hope that this book will make the beginning easier.

# Case 1

# Weakness of the Right Arm and Leg and Numbness of the Left Arm and Leg

# Case 1

A 33-year-old right-handed man with a history of Hodgkin's disease in remission came to the clinic complaining of trouble using his right hand. His symptoms began 4 weeks previously and had gradually worsened. He found it difficult to open jar lids and occasionally dropped objects from his right hand, but he was able to reach up for objects on high shelves without difficulty. The left leg, and later the left hand, had become numb, described as being similar to the facial sensation that accompanies dental anesthesia. The patient stated that other people had remarked that he dragged his right leg when he walked, and he had experienced difficulty going up stairs. In addition, he had noticed some aching pain over the posterior aspect of the neck.

On examination the patient was alert, oriented, and cooperative. His speech was well articulated and fluent. Naming, repetition, and comprehension were normal. Cranial nerve functions were normal. Proprioception and vibratory sensation were decreased in the right toes, ankle, and fingers. Pinprick and temperature sensation was decreased on the left arm, trunk, and leg, but not on the neck or face. There was normal resistance to passive movement of the right arm and leg (i.e., tone). Mild weakness without wasting or fasciculation was present in the right arm and leg. Specifically, grip was weaker in the right hand than in the left, as was finger abduction. Elbow flexion and extension were normal, as was shoulder abduction. In the right lower extremity, hip flexion and ankle dorsiflexion were weak. Tendon reflexes were increased on the right side, and Babinski's sign was present on that side.

Figure 1-1 represents the cross-sectional anatomy of the nervous system at various levels. The reader should use the figures in this book to draw in the pathways of the different functional systems involved in producing the patient's symptoms and signs. This exercise will aid in understanding how an anatomic diagnosis is constructed. Begin by considering this patient's weakness of the right arm and leg. What functional systems are involved? What are the anatomic distributions of the functional systems?

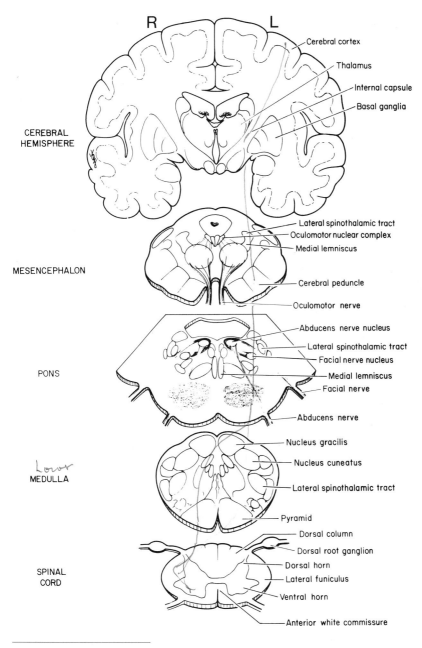

FIGURE 1-1.

# Case 1

The presence of hyperreflexia and Babinski's sign implies an upper motoneuron lesion (lesion of the corticospinal, or pyramidal, system) as the cause of weakness. Muscle tone is measured by the resistance of the patient's limb to passive movement and is increased in patients with lesions of the corticospinal system (especially those lesions of long duration). This increased tone is due to increased excitability of the alpha motoneuron resulting from a release from inhibition. The release from inhibition (disinhibition) of the alpha motoneuron also results in increased excitability of the reflex loop involved in the tendon reflexes; hence, hyperreflexia. Disinhibition also unmasks other reflexes, such as Babinski's sign.

An intact alpha motoneuron and peripheral motor nerve are required for reflexes. The presence of the reflexes in this case implies that the alpha motoneurons and the peripheral motor nerve are intact. If they were involved, one would see hyporeflexia and hypotonia in addition to weakness. Disorders of the muscle or neuromuscular junction usually do not alter reflexes or tone. Lesions of the alpha motoneuron can usually be differentiated from lesions of the peripheral motor nerve by the presence of fasciculations in alpha motoneuron disease.

Figure 1-2 is a representation of a series of sections through the CNS. The pathway of the corticospinal system carrying the upper motoneuron is traced by the solid line. The involved corticospinal system arises from areas 4 and 6 of the left frontal lobe. It descends in the left cerebral peduncle of the midbrain and then in the left basis pontis. Next it crosses to the opposite side in the pyramids of the medulla to descend in the right lateral funiculus of the spinal cord. Finally, the corticospinal fibers synapse in the ventral horn of the spinal cord.

A lesion anywhere along this pathway at or above the fourth cervical spinal cord level (C4) could cause the patient's symptoms of right-sided weakness. The lesion has to be above the C5 level. Since the biceps is innervated by the C5 and C6 segments, a lesion at the C5 level would cause the right biceps tendon reflex to be decreased. The increased activity of this reflex implies that the corticospinal fibers are involved above this level.

More information is needed to determine the precise anatomic site of the lesion. Further information can be obtained from analysis of other symptoms and signs. Consider next what system is responsible for the patient's decreased perception of pinprick on the left side. The reader may wish to sketch the pathway of the system(s) on Figure 1-2.

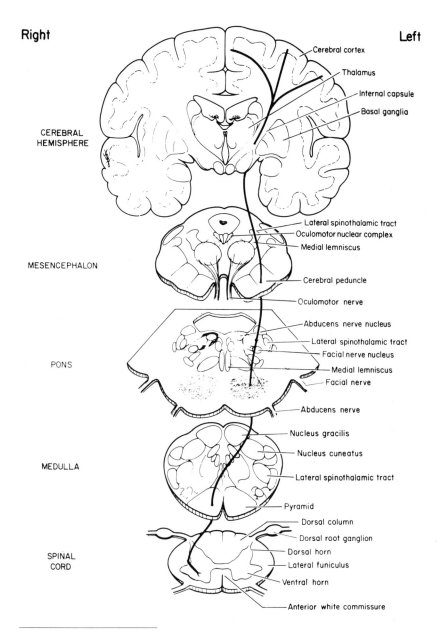

FIGURE 1.2.
Solid line: corticospinal tract.

The symptom of numbness in the left upper and lower extremities suggests involvement of the spinothalamic system. This is confirmed by the absence of pinprick and temperature sensation found on examination. The other major pathway subserving sensation, the dorsal column or medial lemniscal system, mediates discriminative sensations such as proprioception and vibration. With lesions of this system the patient may complain that the limb feels heavy or is clumsy in use. To Figure 1-2 has been added the pathway of the spinothalamic tract (dashed line, Fig. 1-3). The first-order neuron with its cell body in the dorsal root ganglion enters the spinal cord via the dorsal root. The first-order neuron synapses on the second-order neuron in the dorsal horn of the spinal cord. This neuron then crosses to the other side of the spinal cord through the anterior white commissure. It ascends in the lateral funiculus to synapse in the ventral posterior lateral nucleus of thalamus. From there, the third-order neuron ascends to the somatosensory area of the cerebral cortex.

At this point it can be seen that the only anatomic site where a single small lesion can affect both the corticospinal and spinothalamic systems is on the right side below the pyramidal decussation but above the C5 level of the spinal cord.

In the spinal cord the ascending fibers are laminated such that the fibers entering from the lower levels are more lateral and superficial. Therefore, these fibers are more vulnerable to compression by an extrinsic lesion. As the lesion expands, more fibers are involved and the sensory symptoms appear to ascend. Fibers of the corticospinal system are similarly laminated, and progressive spinal cord compression can cause an ascending pattern of weakness. This ascending picture secondary to spinal cord compression is sometimes confused with a similar complaint in Guillain-Barré syndrome. This illustrates an important principle: The level of a spinal cord lesion suggested by the history and examination suggests only the lower limit of the lesion.

**D**oes this lesion also explain why the patient had decreased vibratory and proprioceptive sensations on the right side? What functional systems mediate vibration and proprioception?

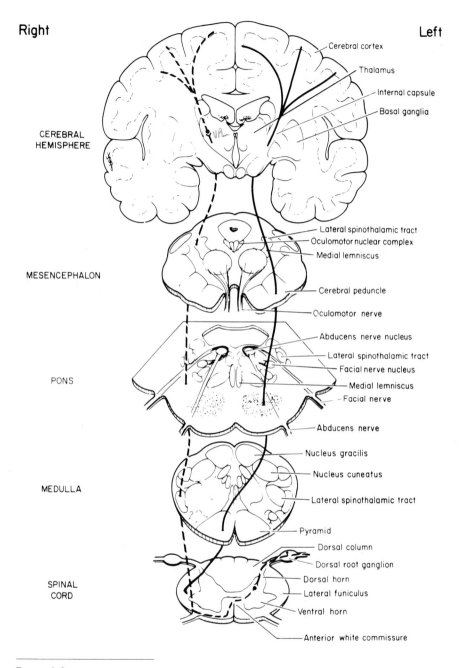

FIGURE 1-3.
Solid line: corticospinal tract; dashed line: lateral spinothalamic tract.

Vibratory and proprioceptive sensations are mediated by the dorsal column or medial lemniscal system, which is traced by the dotted line in Figure 1-4. The first-order neuron, whose cell body is in the dorsal root ganglion, enters the spinal cord via the dorsal root. It ascends in the ipsilateral dorsal column of the spinal cord without synapsing or crossing to the other side. In the medulla, first-order neurons synapse in the nucleus gracilis from spinal segments below T6, while those from more rostral spinal segments synapse in the nucleus cuneatus. Here, the second-order neuron axons cross to the other side to form the medial lemniscus. These fibers then ascend to synapse on the third-order neurons in the thalamus. These thalamic neuron axons ascend to somatosensory areas of the parietal lobe cortex.

From examination of Figure 1-4, in which the involved medial lemniscal system has been added to the previous figure, which contained the involved corticospinal and spinothalamic pathways, one can see that the proposed spinal cord lesion, besides accounting for the patient's right-sided weakness and left-sided loss of pinprick sensation, also explains the right-sided loss of vibratory and proprioceptive sensation. These symptoms and signs of a hemispinal cord lesion (lesion of one-half of the spinal cord) are known as the Brown-Séquard syndrome.

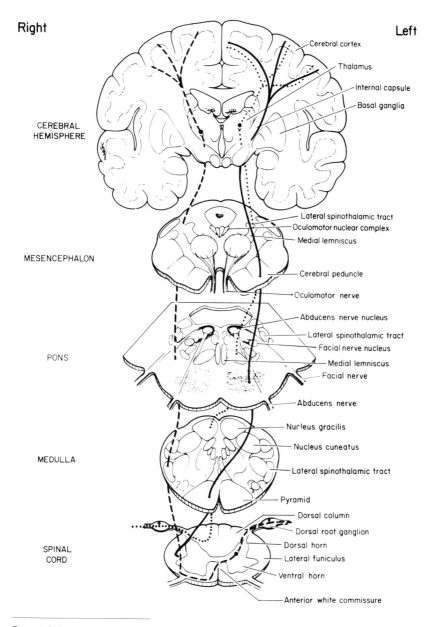

FIGURE 1-4.
Solid line: corticospinal tract; dashed line: lateral spinothalamic tract; dotted line: medial lemniscus.

Once the anatomic diagnosis has been defined, the next step is to formulate a pathologic differential diagnosis (Fig. 1-5). Some possibilities are determined by pathologic alterations of tissues already present at the anatomic site. Meninges surrounding the spinal cord can give rise to meningiomas. Astrocytes and ependymal cells in the spinal cord can give rise to astrocytomas and ependymomas, respectively. Schwannomas and neurofibromas arising from the Schwann cells in the spinal roots can compress the spinal cord. Vascular occlusion, spinal cord hemorrhages, or epidural hematomas (especially in patients with bleeding disorders) are less likely to cause a lesion restricted to one-half of the spinal cord, but these possibilities do exist. Other types of pathology not arising from tissue normally present may still occur in this region and must be included in the pathologic differential diagnosis—for example, metastatic cancer.

The list of pathologic possibilities may be quite lengthy. This list can be reduced to a manageable number by ordering the pathologic differential diagnoses according to their probability (Fig. 1-5), as determined by review of the history and physical examination findings. The most probable possibilities in the pathologic differential diagnosis become the neurologic differential diagnosis.

In the case presented, symptoms progressed over a 4-week period, suggesting a slowly expanding lesion, such as a tumor. As already noted, the history of an ascending motor loss is suggestive of an extrinsic lesion compressing the spinal cord. This makes tumors arising from within the spinal cord less likely. Therefore, tumors such as meningiomas, schwannomas, neurofibromas, or metastases are more likely. Since the patient has a history of Hodgkin's disease, the most likely possibility is that of spinal cord compression from a lymphoma. The patient was found on myelography to have spinal cord compression at C3 consistent with Hodgkin's lymphoma. The patient underwent radiation therapy and had resolution of his symptoms and signs.

A final note: Seldom is the lesion confined to only one-half of the spinal cord. This is particularly true of tumors compressing the spinal cord. However, symptoms and signs of a spinal cord lesion are often asymmetrical. The greater loss of strength on one side and of pinprick sensation on the other side is highly suggestive of a spinal cord lesion because of the anatomic principles outlined above.

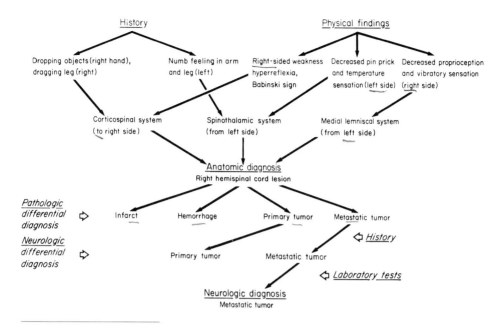

FIGURE 1-5.

**Case 2**

# Right-Sided Weakness and Left Gaze Paresis

*Foville's syndrome*
*Left pontine Lesion*

# Case 2

A 60-year-old right-handed man was brought to the emergency room by his family because of the sudden onset of difficulty in walking. He had been in his usual state of good health until that morning, when he fell while trying to get out of bed. He was able to get back up but later dragged his right leg while walking. He found that his right upper extremity was weak when he tried to grasp objects for support. His family noted that he was drooling from the left side of his mouth. The patient understood what people said to him, but the family thought that his speech was slurred. He denied double vision, loss of vision, or any change in sensation.

On neurologic examination the patient was alert, oriented and cooperative. His speech was slurred but fluent, without word-finding difficulty. Speech and reading comprehension were normal. The pupils were 3 mm in diameter and reactive to light. On command, the patient could look conjugately to the right, up, and down, but not to the left (i.e., he had a left gaze paresis). Visual fields were intact to confrontation. When he spoke, the left side of his face did not move. When he was asked to smile, the right side moved appropriately while the left side remained immobile. When he attempted to close his eyes tight the left eyelashes could easily be seen, while the lashes on the right were buried. The wrinkles of the left side of the forehead were less pronounced. The tongue protruded in the midline, and the palate was elevated in the midline. Pinprick, light touch, proprioceptive, and vibratory sensations were intact. There were hyperreflexia and weakness of the right extremities. Babinski's sign was present on the right. The finger-to-nose test (in which the patient alternately moves his index finger between the examiner's index finger and the patient's own nose) was performed without ataxia or tremor on the left side, but the patient was unable to perform the task on the right. The right upper extremity was slightly flexed at the elbow, and the slightly extended right lower extremity moved slowly and stiffly when the patient attempted to walk.

Consider the patient's right-sided weakness: The involvement of what system accounts for such weakness, and what is the anatomy of that system? The reader may wish to draw the system on Figure 2-1.

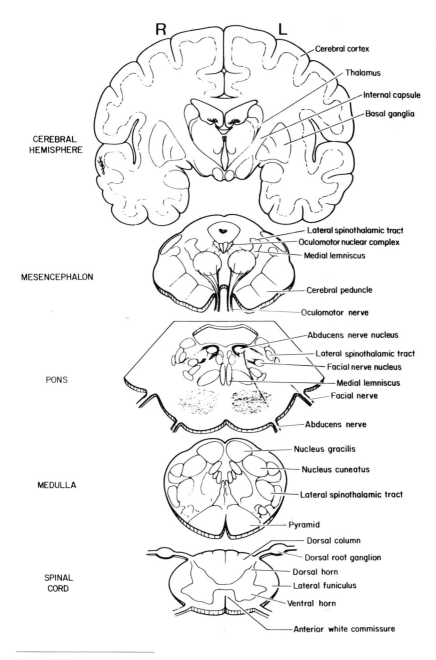

FIGURE 2-1.

## Case 2

Hyperreflexia and Babinski's sign on the right imply that his weakness is caused by a lesion of the corticospinal system. Its pathway through the CNS is traced in Figure 2-2 by the solid line. The abnormalities of the patient's gait are consistent with an upper motoneuron lesion and are those of a hemiparetic gait.

The upper motoneuron, or corticospinal pathway, runs the entire length of the CNS. Since the muscles of the upper extremity are innervated by the C4–T1 spinal cord segments, a lesion anywhere along this pathway above the C4 spinal cord level could cause weakness of the right extremities. The hyperreflexic right biceps tendon reflex suggests that the corticospinal fibers to the anterior horn cells supplying the biceps must be affected. The anterior horn cells to the biceps lie at the C5 and C6 levels. Therefore, evaluation of the tendon reflex abnormalities and the corticospinal system indicates that the lesion must be at or above the C4 level.

More information is needed to arrive at the specific anatomic site of the lesion. Where is the lesion producing the paralysis of the upper and lower face on the left?

The most likely cause of the facial weakness is damage to either the upper motoneuron, facial nucleus, or facial nerve fasciculus, since the involvement of the corticospinal tract, as previously discussed, suggests that the lesion is within the CNS. This consideration excludes peripheral nerve, neuromuscular junction, or muscle as the locus of the lesion causing the facial weakness. A knowledge of the unique anatomy of cortical projections to the facial nerve nucleus allows one to decide between an upper motoneuron lesion and a lower motoneuron lesion. Decide which is involved and consider the anatomy.

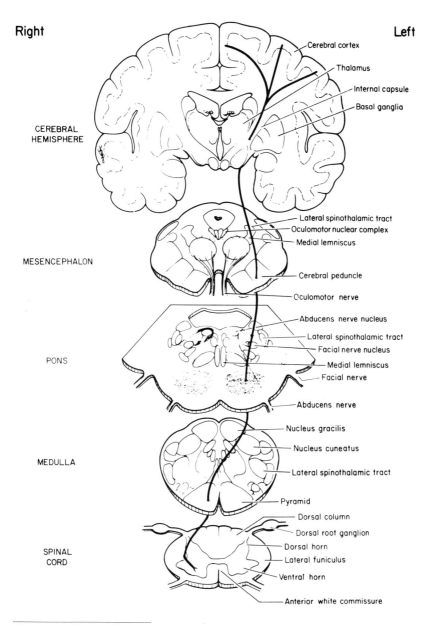

FIGURE 2-2.
Solid line: corticospinal tract.

Each facial nerve nucleus can be functionally divided into two regions, one that supplies the muscles of the upper face and the other, the lower face. It is thought that these two divisions differ in their upper motoneuron input: The part of the facial nerve nucleus that supplies the muscles of the upper part of the face receives input from both cerebral hemispheres (Fig. 2-3A, B), while that part of the facial nerve nucleus supplying the lower part of the face receives only contralateral input. Therefore, a lower motoneuron lesion (i.e., of the nucleus itself) or a lesion of the peripheral nerve would result in a loss of innervation to both the upper and lower face (represented by the broken lines in Fig. 2-3A). The patient would be unable to move either the upper or lower part of the face. This is called a lower motoneuron or peripheral type of facial weakness. A lesion of the contralateral hemisphere would result in a loss of innervation to the part of the nucleus sending fibers to the lower face (see the broken line in Fig. 2-3B). The part of the nucleus sending fibers to the upper face would continue to be innervated by the intact ipsilateral hemisphere (solid line in Fig. 2-3B). In this case the patient would be able to move the upper part of the face but not the lower part. This is called the upper motoneuron or central type of facial weakness.

In the setting of an acute lesion of corticobulbar fibers to the facial nucleus, the ipsilateral innervation to the facial nerve nucleus from the intact hemisphere may not be able to compensate completely. For a few hours to days the upper face may also be mildly weak, and, therefore, the condition may resemble a lower motoneuron facial weakness. However, the upper face usually regains its strength. Cautious interpretation is necessary in the acute situation.

Careful testing of facial function is required. Some patients with an upper motoneuron or central facial weakness may have a symmetrical smile in response to a joke, whereas the face is asymmetrical when the person is asked to smile volitionally. This demonstrates that structures other than the corticospinal system can generate movement. Indeed, these other structures may account for recovery of function following a lesion of the corticospinal system. With slowly progressive lesions of the motor cortex or with recovery, the only remaining deficit may be limited to decreased dexterity of the fingers of the involved hand.

In the present case there was a paralysis of the upper and lower face on the left. What is the anatomic lesion underlying this sign?

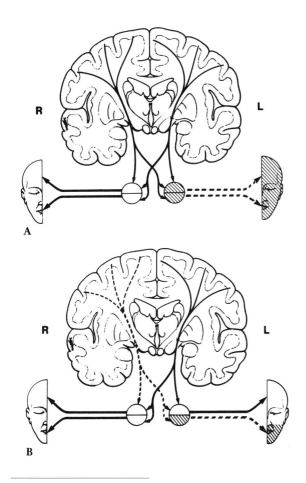

FIGURE 2-3.

## Case 2

The patient has involvement of both the upper and lower face. Therefore, a lesion of the facial nucleus or fasciculus (the portion of the facial nerve axons within the brainstem) is present. Superimposing this lesion on the illustration of CNS anatomy (broken line in Fig. 2-4) demonstrates that a lesion in the left side of the pons explains both the patient's left facial weakness and the right arm and leg weakness. Patients with facial weakness may have slurred speech, as in this case. Certain sounds like "me" or "pa" require closure of the obicularis oris and, therefore, may be distorted when facial nerve lesions are present.

The clinical picture apparent thus far is that of a "crossed paralysis," in which there are paralysis or weakness of one side of the body and a cranial nerve weakness, in this case on the other side of the body (face). This pattern is specific to brainstem lesions and should alert the examiner to this possibility.

Does this proposed lesion in the left pons explain the patient's inability to move his eyes fully to the left?

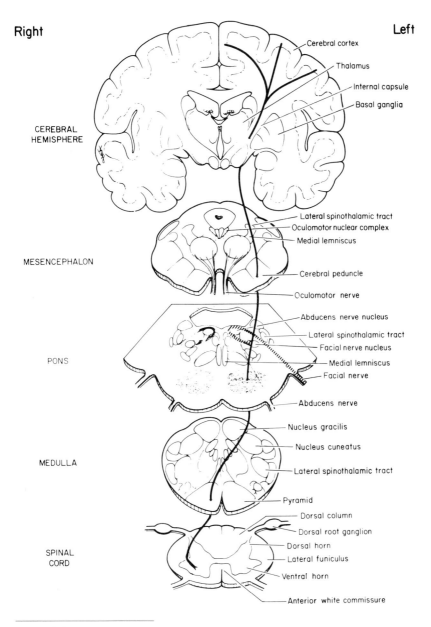

FIGURE 2-4.
Solid line: corticospinal tract; broken line: facial nerve.

**Case 2**

The system involved in moving the eyes conjugately to the left originates in the right frontal eye field (area 8) of the cerebral cortex (Fig. 2-5). Fibers descend from the right frontal eye field through the internal capsule to the right side of the midbrain. Here, fibers cross to the left side at the level of the lower midbrain. These fibers then descend to the lower pontine level and synapse in an area called the paramedian pontine reticular formation (PPRF). Fibers then leave the PPRF and synapse in the ipsilateral (in this case, left) abducens nucleus. There are two populations of neurons in the abducens nucleus: motoneurons, which run to the lateral rectus muscle to abduct the ipsilateral eye, and interneurons, which cross the midline at the level of the abducens nucleus to ascend in the contralateral medial longitudinal fasciculus (MLF) and synapse in the medial rectus subnucleus of the oculomotor nucleus. Therefore, when the PPRF activates the abducens nucleus, the eyes move conjugately to the ipsilateral side by innervating the ipsilateral lateral rectus and contralateral medial rectus muscles. A lesion of the PPRF or closely adjacent abducens nucleus, therefore, produces a horizontal gaze palsy when the patient attempts to look toward the side of the lesion, as in this case. A lesion above the lower midbrain of the descending fibers from the right frontal eye field causes loss of voluntary gaze toward the contralateral side. A lesion of this pathway below the lower midbrain causes the loss of conjugate volitional gaze toward the ipsilateral side.

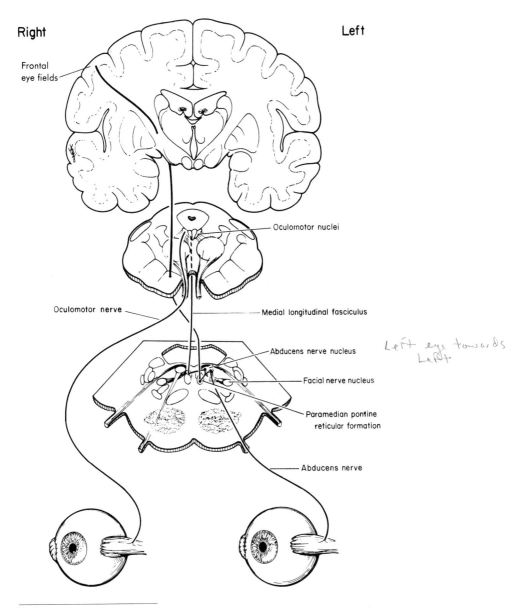

FIGURE 2-5.

Case 2

Consider the anatomy of the three involved systems discussed so far (Fig. 2-6). The anatomic diagnosis is a left pontine lesion. This is the only site where one lesion could explain all the patient's symptoms and signs. This constellation of findings is known as Foville's syndrome.

Due to the limited response of nervous tissue to injury, analysis of the neurologic deficits yields only the anatomic diagnosis. A stroke causes the same hemiparesis as does a tumor or abscess. However, the history of these different types of pathologic process does vary. Strokes are of sudden onset. Tumors tend to develop more slowly, although infrequently they also present suddenly, with or without seizures. The newcomer is advised first to think broadly concerning the pathologic possibilities. Then careful reflection on the history and physical findings will allow the selection of the most likely possibilities.

A variety of pathologic lesions may affect this anatomic site. Tumors, abscesses, hemorrhage, and occlusions of blood vessels are some of the possibilities in the pathologic differential diagnosis. However, when there is a history of a sudden onset, as in this case, the most probable pathologic possibility is infarction or hemorrhage. These constitute the neurologic differential diagnosis. No hemorrhage was seen on the CT scan, and the neurologic diagnosis is, therefore, an infarct of the left pons.

---

*Handwritten notes:*

Left pontine lesion

a) Left gaze paresis
b) Left face weakness (upper MN)
c) Rt arm weakness
d) Rt leg weakness

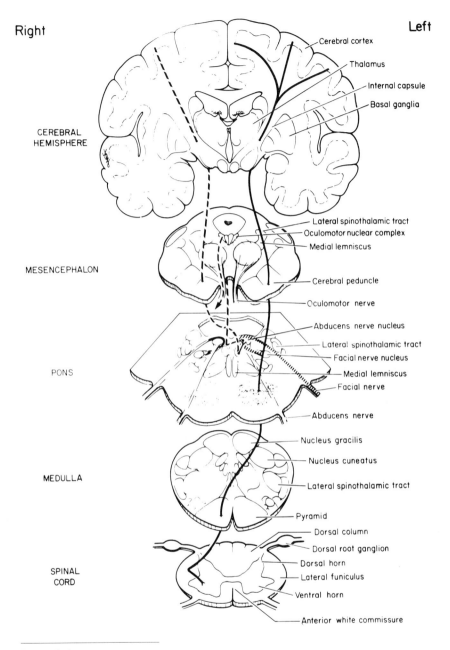

FIGURE 2-6.
Solid line: corticospinal tract; dashed line: corticobulbar fibers to PPRF.

# Case 3

# Right-Sided Weakness and Double Vision

## Case 3

**A** 73-year-old right-handed man was brought into the emergency room because he was unable to walk. Several weeks previously he noticed that he was dragging his right leg while walking. He had to lean on a chair to stand, and he pushed the chair around in order to walk. When the right leg became so weak that he could not get out of bed, he allowed his daughter to bring him to the emergency room. During this same period of time the right upper extremity also became increasingly weak. He would drop objects from the right hand and he was unable to raise the right hand above his head. Further, over this period the patient noted drooping of the left eyelid. By the time he finally came to the emergency room the left eye was completely closed. The patient observed that if he manually lifted the left eyelid, he saw double, with the two images perceived as being oblique to each other.

**T**he patient was alert, oriented, and cooperative. His speech was well articulated and fluent. Naming, repetition, and comprehension were normal. Visual fields were full to confrontation. The right pupil was 3 mm in diameter and reacted normally to light. The left pupil was 7 mm and unreactive to light. The patient could not adduct, elevate, or depress the left eye; however, abduction was full. Attempts to look down resulted in counterclockwise rotation of the left eye. Right eye movements were full. A complete left ptosis (i.e., drooping of the left eyelid) was noted. The lower portion of the right side of the face did not move as well as the left, but both sides of the forehead wrinkled well. Pinprick, proprioceptive, and vibratory sensations remained normal. There was marked weakness with increased muscle tone and hyperreflexia in the right upper and lower extremities. A right-sided Babinski's sign was found. On the finger-to-nose test there was no ataxia or tremor on the left side. The patient could not perform this test with the right arm because he could not raise it off the bed sufficiently. He was unable to support his weight with his right leg and thus was unable to walk.

**W**hat functional system is involved to account for the right-sided weakness? What is the anatomy of that system? What does this imply about the anatomic diagnosis? The reader may wish to trace the anatomy of the involved system on Figure 3-1.

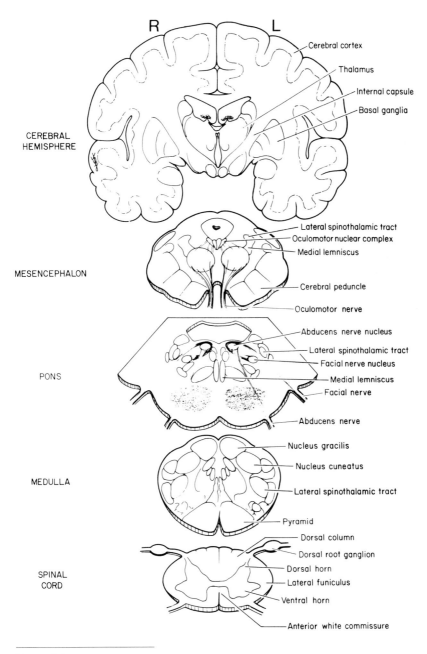

FIGURE 3-1.

The weakness, increased tone, Babinski's sign, and hyperreflexia on the right side imply a lesion of the corticospinal system on the left side above the pyramidal decussation or on the right side below the decussation (traced by a solid line in Fig. 3-2). A lesion anywhere along this pathway at or above the C4 level could result in the patient's right-sided weakness.

More data are needed to refine the anatomic diagnosis. How does an analysis of the facial weakness help to determine this diagnosis?

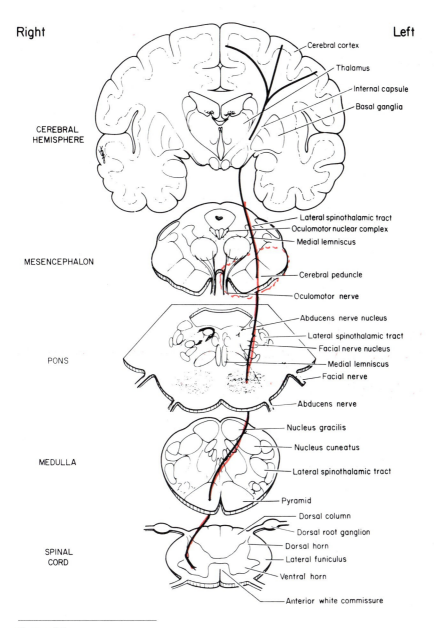

FIGURE 3-2.
Solid line: corticospinal tract.

# Case 3

As discussed previously (see page 28), a lesion of the upper motoneuron to the right facial nucleus is responsible for weakness that affects only the right lower half of the face. A lesion of the nucleus (lower motoneuron) or peripheral nerve would cause weakness of both the upper and lower face. Examination of the pathway of the upper motoneuron from the left cerebral hemisphere to the right facial nucleus (dashed line, Fig. 3-3) and the corticospinal pathway mediating the right-sided weakness (solid line, Fig. 3-3) shows that the lesion had to be on the left side at or above the level of the lower pons.

To localize the anatomic diagnosis to either the cerebral hemisphere, midbrain, or upper pons, next analyze the eye findings. Double vision (diplopia) results from misalignment of the eyes causing a disparity between the relative position of the images on the two retinas. Different patterns of extraocular muscle weakness determine the type of retinal disparity and thus the nature of the diplopia. For example, horizontal diplopia results from weakness of muscles controlling horizontal eye movements, regardless of whether the weakness is due to disorders of the muscle, neuromuscular junction, or nerve.

Determine which extraocular muscles are involved to produce this patient's diplopia. Next, determine which functional anatomic system controls these muscles.

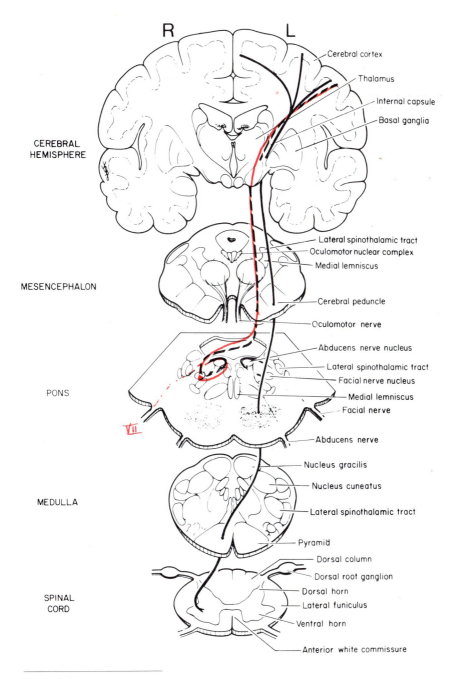

FIGURE 3-3.
Solid line: corticospinal tract; dashed line: corticobulbar fibers to facial nucleus.

# Case 3

The patient cannot adduct, elevate, or depress the left eye. This is explained by weakness of the medial rectus, superior rectus, inferior oblique, and inferior rectus. Intorsion and extorsion are rotatory movements of the globes. Intorsion is the primary action of the superior oblique. When the patient looked down and in, intorsion was observed, implying preserved function of the superior oblique muscle, which is innervated by the trochlear nerve. Full abduction in the left eye denotes sparing of the abducens nerve and lateral rectus muscle.

The oculomotor nerve innervates the medial, inferior, and superior recti and the inferior oblique. Therefore, involvement of this nerve explains the eye muscle weakness (dotted line in Fig. 3-4). Are the other eye findings (pupillary light reflex and left ptosis) consistent with this anatomic diagnosis? The efferent limb of the light reflex runs in the oculomotor nerve, as does the innervation of the levator palpebrae muscle (eyelid elevator). The patient's unreactive pupil and ptosis can also be explained by a lesion of the oculomotor nerve.

As can be seen when the left oculomotor nerve is superimposed on the series of CNS cross sections containing the tracings of the corticospinal and corticobulbar systems (Fig. 3-4), these different systems converge in the left half of the mesencephalon (midbrain). This is the anatomic diagnosis. This constellation of findings is known as Weber's syndrome.

Next, the pathologic differential diagnosis is derived from the anatomic diagnosis. Blood vessels in this region are prone to occlusion or hemorrhage resulting in stroke. Tumors, such as astrocytomas, may arise from tissue normally present. Tumors may also come from metastatic tissue deposited in this region. Other pathologic processes may occur in this region, such as abscesses and demyelination. These pathologic possibilities constitute the pathologic differential diagnosis.

Based on the findings from the history and physical examination and the pathologic differential diagnosis, what is the neurologic differential diagnosis? The gradual onset of symptoms implicates tumor, abscess, inflammatory disorder, or demyelination as the cause of the patient's symptoms. The neurologic differential diagnosis is therefore (1) tumor, (2) abscess or other inflammation, or (3) demyelination. Elevated protein with no white blood cells was found on examination of the cerebrospinal fluid. A CT scan of this patient showed a mass with homogeneous contrast enhancement more characteristic of tumor than of abscess in the left cerebral peduncle. Our neurologic diagnosis is a tumor of the left cerebral peduncle.

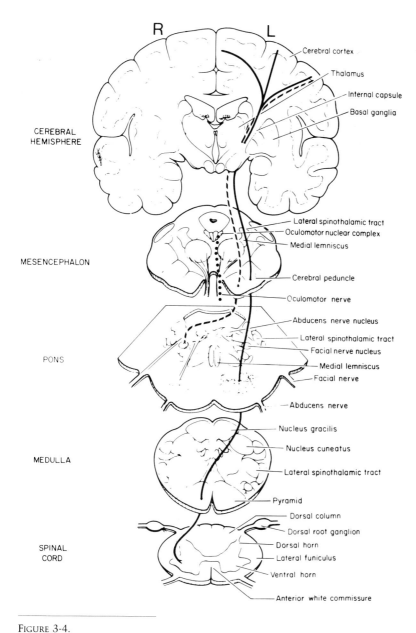

FIGURE 3-4.
Solid line: corticospinal tract; dashed line: corticobulbar fibers to facial nucleus; dotted line: oculomotor nerve.

# Case 4

## Weakness of Both Lower Extremities

? Tumor along midline of motor cortex affecting Upper M.N. for Legs

# Case 4

A 45-year-old woman came to the clinic complaining of weakness of both lower extremities. The weakness was described as stiffness and a tendency to drag her feet while walking. She had to pull herself up stairs using the hand rails. The weakness was first noticed 8 weeks previously and had progressively worsened. Her only other complaint was an intermittent headache. This headache worsened with coughing or bending, and it awakened her from sleep. She denied changes in vision, sensation, coordination, or speech.

The patient was alert and cooperative. Speech was well articulated and fluent. Comprehension was intact. Cranial nerve examination was normal except for papilledema. Sensory examination showed normal vibratory function, proprioception, and responses to pinprick and double simultaneous stimulation. Strength, muscle tone, and dexterity were normal in the upper extremities. When the lower extremities were examined, there was moderate weakness, hypertonia, and hyperreflexia. Babinski's signs were present bilaterally.

Consider the weakness in the lower extremities. What system(s) is (are) involved to produce the patient's weakness? Where is the lesion along the anatomic pathway of the involved system(s)? The reader may wish to sketch in the involved system(s) on Fig. 4-1.

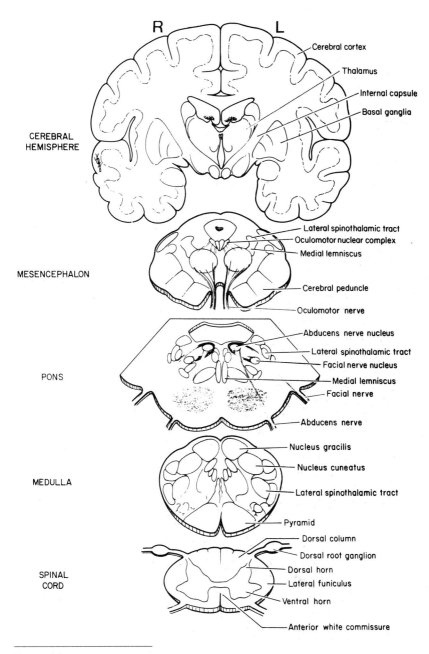

FIGURE 4-1.

Increased tone, hyperreflexia, and Babinski's signs mean that the lesion involves the upper motoneuron in its course through the corticospinal system (the solid line in Fig. 4-2). The pathway to the left leg follows the same course on the opposite side (Fig. 4-2, broken line). The anatomic lesion must be situated so as to affect both right and left descending corticospinal pathways to the lower extremities while sparing those to the upper extremities.

From Figure 4-2 one might propose the medullary decussation as the anatomic site, which would involve corticospinal fibers to the lower extremities bilaterally. However, corticospinal fibers for the upper extremities run in the same small area. It is highly improbable that a lesion here would affect only those corticospinal fibers to the legs, sparing those to the arms. A spinal cord lesion affecting the corticospinal tract below the T1 level would affect both lower extremities but spare the upper extremities. However, it is unlikely that a spinal cord lesion would completely spare the dorsal column systems or spinothalamic sensory systems.

Where is the patient's lesion?

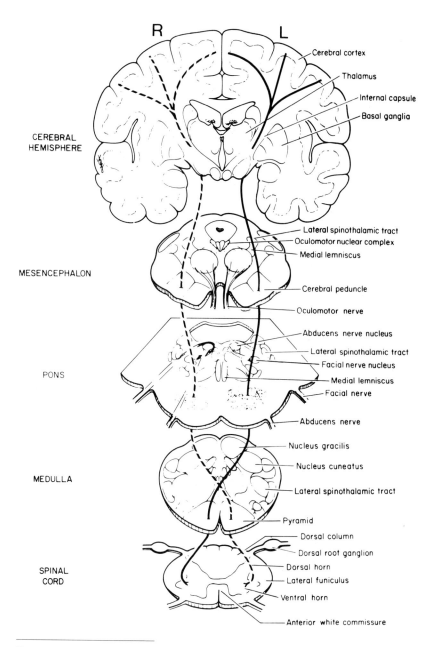

FIGURE 4-2.
Solid and dashed lines: corticospinal tracts.

The origins of the corticospinal fibers are spread out over the motor strip of the cerebral cortex (Fig. 4-3). The corticospinal fibers to the legs originate in the medial convexity of the cerebral hemisphere, whereas those to the arms and face come from the lateral convexities. By the time corticospinal fibers originating in the cerebral cortex reach the internal capsule, they are well mixed. Lesions involving the corticospinal system at this level usually produce weakness in both the upper and lower extremities. Lesions in the brainstem affecting the corticospinal fibers act similarly. In the spinal cord the fibers are organized in a laminar function so that fibers to the lower extremities may be affected but not those to the upper extremities (see case 1). Therefore, a midline lesion affecting the medial convexities of both cerebral hemispheres, while sparing the lateral convexities, is most likely. Such a lesion would affect only the origins of the corticospinal fibers to the leg, sparing those to the arm and face. Furthermore, a midline lesion anterior to the parietal lobes would spare sensation. This anatomic diagnosis would explain the patient's clinical presentation.

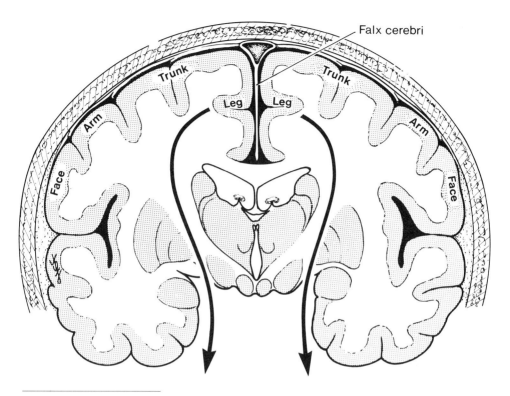

FIGURE 4-3.

After identifying the anatomic site, the neurologist then formulates a pathologic differential diagnosis. Here again, a knowledge of the structures and tissues present at this site aids in developing the pathologic differential diagnosis.

At the vertex of the skull, primary or metastatic tumors or a depressed fracture could compromise the medial convexities of the cerebral hemispheres. In the epidural and subdural spaces are blood vessels, which, when ruptured, cause hematomas. Meningiomas may arise from meninges at this site. Meningiomas of the falx cerebri may compress leg areas of the adjacent motor cortex. Infarction of a single anterior cerebral artery supplying both medial convexities could result in bilateral leg weakness. Corticospinal fibers to the lower extremities run adjacent to the bodies of the lateral ventricles. Sudden enlargement of these ventricles (hydrocephalus) may stretch these fibers, producing leg weakness.

The pathologic differential diagnosis can be quite long. It is reduced by considering ancillary findings on history and physical examination. The patient's history of headache implies possible increased intracranial pressure. This is further supported by the examiner's observations of papilledema and the patient's report of headaches worsened by coughing and bending over, which act to increase intrathoracic and intraabdominal pressure. This results in increased venous pressure, which is transmitted via the internal jugular vein (does not contain valves) to the cranial cavity, exaggerating the intracranial pressure. The gradual progression of symptoms also is consistent with an expanding lesion.

Order the pathologic differential diagnosis for this case according to probability and thus formulate the neurologic differential diagnosis.

A meningioma of the falx cerebri is the most likely diagnosis (Fig. 4-4). Such tumors occur more often in women. There is no history of symptoms suggesting subarachnoid hemorrhage (i.e., abrupt headache, neck stiffness, depressed level of consciousness), which reduces the probability of subarachnoid hemorrhage from rupture of an aneurysm. The absence of head trauma reduces the likelihood of epidural or subdural hematomas. The gradual progression of symptoms virtually precludes an infarction from the neurologic differential diagnosis. A CT scan was performed, and a mass arising from the falx was confirmed. A meningioma was removed at operation.

If this were a case of a 65-year-old woman who struck her head in a fall two weeks previously, what would be the most likely item in the neurologic differential diagnosis?

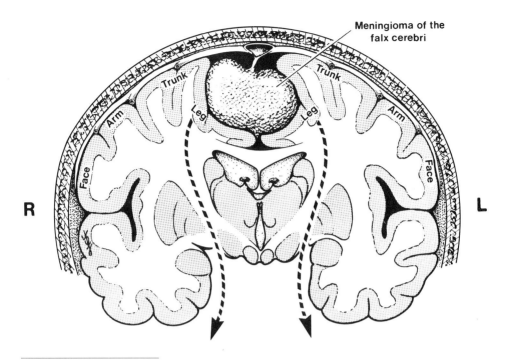

FIGURE 4-4.

The clinical presentation again is that of a lesion in the region of the medial convexities of the cerebral hemisphere. The history of gradual progression and headaches implies an expanding mass lesion causing increased intracranial pressure. The pathologic differential diagnosis would still include the possibility of a meningioma arising from the falx cerebri. However, the history of head trauma suggests that other possibilities in the pathologic differential diagnosis are more probable. Intracranial hematomas may result from head trauma. These hematomas are intraparenchymal, subdural, or epidural. Subdural hematomas can occur bilaterally over the medial cerebral convexities. A subdural (parasagittal subdural) hematoma would be most consistent with this patient's clinical presentation.

Again, a knowledge of neuroanatomy can explain why these hematomas are likely to occur in the parasagittal region. The cortical veins drain the surface of the brain and empty into the superior sagittal sinus (Fig. 4-5A, B). When the patient fell and struck her head, the moving skull came to a sudden stop while the brain continued forward. This movement produced a shearing force on the bridging cortical veins, which at one end were moving with the brain and on the other end were fixed to the stationary skull. The veins ruptured at the attachment to the superior sagittal sinus (Fig. 4-5B). This bleeding resulted in parasagittal subdural hematomas, which are often bilateral.

The higher incidence of subdural hematomas in the elderly reflects certain anatomic changes that occur with age. With cerebral atrophy, which sometimes accompanies age, there is compensatory enlargement of the subarachnoid space. The brain can then move a greater distance with less severe blows to the head, causing greater shearing of the bridging veins.

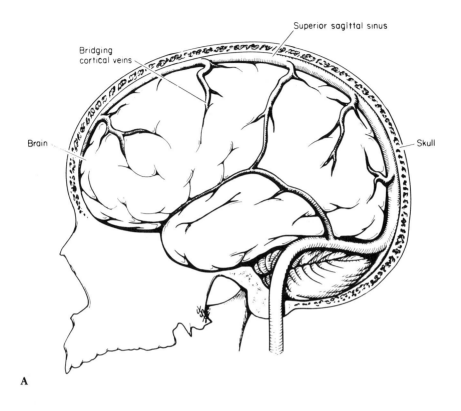

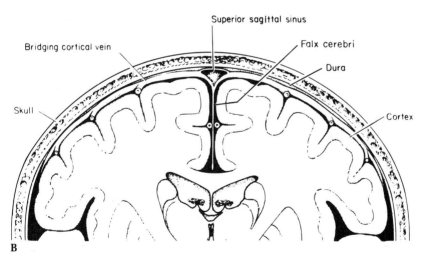

Figure 4-5.

# Case 5

# Dizziness, Ataxia, Right Arm Clumsiness, and Right-Sided Decreased Sensation

*Wallenberg's or Lateral Medullary*

# Case 5

A 58-year-old man was watering his garden when he suddenly noticed that his right arm and hand were clumsy. When he tried to water his plants, the hand and arm holding the hose shook uncontrollably, and he missed his target. The shaking stopped once he put the hose down and rested. He stated that he could still grip the water nozzle strongly. He was unable to tell that the nozzle felt cold with his left hand but could with his right hand. At that time, he became nauseated and dizzy, in a manner he described as being similar to the sensation when one spins in a circle a number of times and then stops (ie., vertigo). When he tried to walk, he would stagger, falling toward the right.

In the emergency room his speech was hoarse. While walking, he was ataxic and fell to the right. He was equally unsteady when he stood with his feet together, with eyes either open or closed (i.e., Romberg's sign was absent). The right eyelid was ptotic, but not completely. Pupil diameter was 2 mm on the right and 5 mm on the left. There was horizontal nystagmus on lateral gaze. He failed to blink with either eye when the right cornea was touched, but both eyes blinked when the left cornea was touched. Pinprick felt less sharp on the right side of the face. Sweating was present only on the left side of the face. The left, but not the right, side of the palate elevated when the posterior wall of the oropharynx was touched with a cotton swab. There was decreased sensation to pinprick and temperature on the left side of the body, but light touch, proprioceptive, and vibratory sensations were normal. The right arm and leg were hypotonic, but strength was normal. The patellar tendon reflex was pendular on the right (i.e., the right leg continued to swing like a pendulum after the patellar tendon had been struck). Movements of the right limbs were dysmetric, and fine motor movements were clumsy.

Begin with the patient's sensory loss. What functional system(s) is (are) associated with this pattern of sensory loss? Note that the patient has "crossed analgesia," with decreased pain sensation on the right side of the face and on the left side of the body. What are the implications of these findings for the anatomic diagnosis?

Figure 5-1 represents the cross-sectional anatomy of the CNS at various levels. To aid in determining the anatomic diagnosis the reader may wish to trace the anatomy of the involved functional system(s).

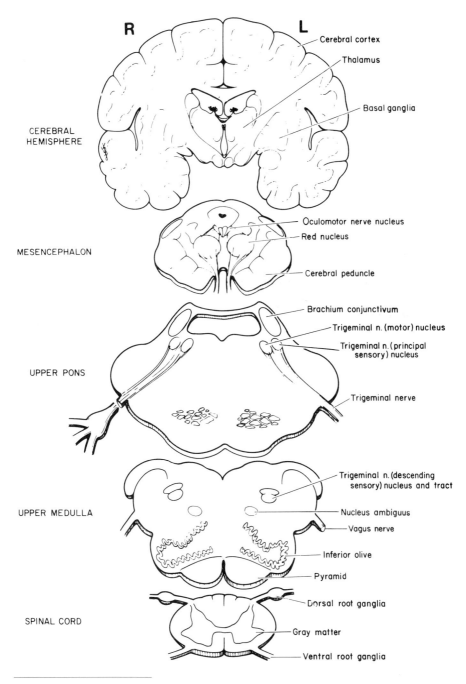

Figure 5-1.

Case 5

Anesthesia of the face is caused by a lesion at one of three levels within the pathway that mediates pain sensation from the right side of the face (solid line, Fig. 5-2). The first-order neuron has its cell body in the trigeminal nerve ganglion. Its dendrites are the sensory receptors, and its axon enters the spinal trigeminal nucleus in the upper pons.

The trigeminal nuclear complex contains four nuclei. The principal sensory nucleus receives tactile information. The mesencephalic nucleus is important for proprioception. The spinal trigeminal nucleus receives pain and temperature sensation input and extends from the upper pons to the C2 level of the spinal cord. Second-order neurons, whose cell bodies lie in the spinal trigeminal nucleus, send their axons crossing to the other side to ascend with the contralateral medial lemniscus (the ventral trigeminal tract) and synapse on the third-order neurons in the thalamus. The third-order neurons send their axons to the somatosensory cortex of the parietal lobe.

A lesion anywhere along this pathway would decrease pain and temperature sensation on the right side of the face. How does the finding of decreased pain and temperature sensation on the left side of the body contribute to the anatomic diagnosis?

The proposed anatomic lesion site would have to affect both the ascending spinothalamic system from the left side of the body (dashed line, Fig. 5-2) and the contralateral trigeminal system. This could occur only with a right-sided lesion between the upper pons and the C2 level of the spinal cord that involves the right descending spinal trigeminal nucleus and the spinothalamic tract. Such a lesion would also explain the loss of the direct corneal reflex on the right side, since the afferent (i.e., sensory) limb of this reflex is mediated by the trigeminal nerve.

Further refinement of the anatomic diagnosis requires more information. Consider the patient's hoarse speech and absent gag reflex on the right. What structure, when lesioned, would cause these symptoms and signs?

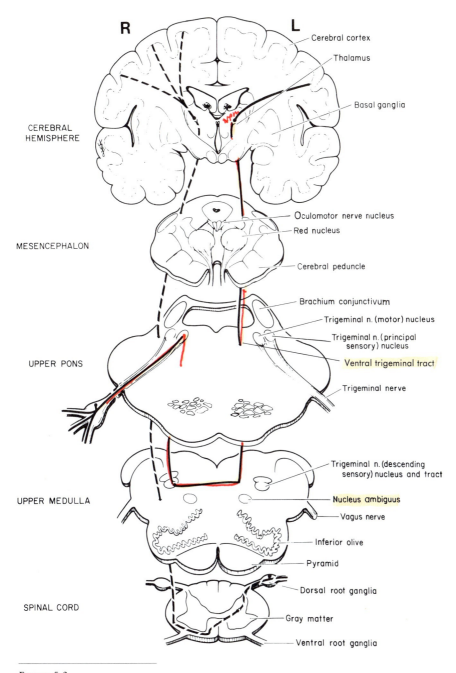

FIGURE 5-2.

Solid line: spinothalamic system from face; dashed line: spinothalamic system from body.

Case 5

Hoarseness implies weakness of one of the vocal cords, which are innervated by the vagus nerve. Vocal cord paralysis is thus caused by lesions of the nucleus ambiguus or of efferent axons coursing through the brainstem to exit with the vagus nerve (dotted line, Fig. 5-3). In addition, testing of the gag reflex showed the right palate to be paralyzed. Other motor axons from the nucleus ambiguus, which course in the glossopharyngeal nerve (not shown in Fig. 5-3), innervate muscles of the larynx, pharynx, and soft palate. A lesion of the right nucleus ambiguus therefore accounts for the patient's hoarseness and his right palate paralysis.

A lesion that involves the nucleus ambiguus and the anatomic site suggested by analysis of the sensory loss imply an anatomic diagnosis in the upper medulla (Fig. 5-3). Is this lesion consistent with other findings? The patient is clumsy on the right, has right-sided ptosis, miosis, and anhydrosis, is vertiginous, and has gaze-evoked horizontal nystagmus.

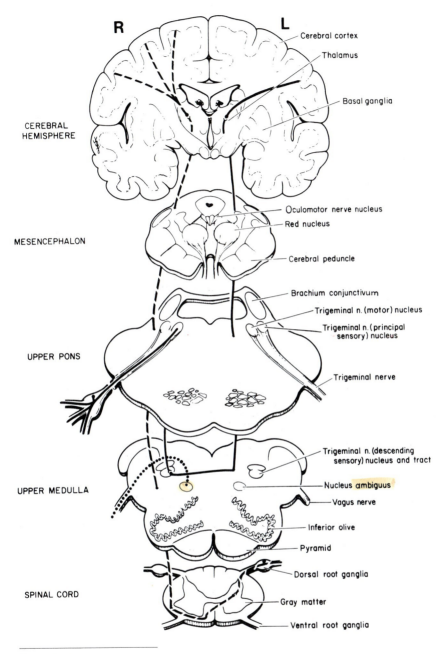

Figure 5-3.
Solid line: spinothalamic system from face; dashed line: spinothalamic system from body; dotted line: vagus nerve.

Clumsiness and incoordination are symptoms associated with position sense loss, weakness, vestibular dysfunction, or cerebellar dysfunction. In the present case, the ataxia, dysmetria, and intention tremor may be explained by lesions of the ipsilateral cerebellum or its efferent or afferent connections. The inferior cerebellar peduncle lies in the upper medulla and carries information to the cerebellum from the vestibular nuclei, the spinal cord, the brainstem reticular formation, and the inferior olivary complex. It also conveys fibers from the cerebellum to the vestibular nuclei and brainstem reticular formation. The symptoms of clumsiness, dyscoordination, and falling to the right coupled with the signs of dysmetria, ataxia, unsteadiness with eyes open on Romberg testing, and hypotonia with pendular reflexes are explained by involvement of the inferior cerebellar peduncle at the level of the upper medulla on the right side.

Vestibular input is conveyed from the labyrinth of the inner ear (vestibular portion of the vestibulocochlear cranial nerve) to the vestibular nucleus in the dorsolateral lower pons and upper medulla. Dysfunction of this system, whether it be peripheral (labyrinthine) or central (vestibulocochlear nerve or vestibular nucleus), causes vertigo with nausea and nystagmus. The vestibular nucleus lies in the lateral brainstem at the level of the lower pons and upper medulla near the descending nucleus and tract of the trigeminal nerve and the lateral spinothalamic tract. A lesion in this area would explain the nystagmus and vertigo.

The Romberg sign is elicited by having a patient stand with his feet together and eyes open. His control of posture and balance is noted, and he is then told to close his eyes. His response is again observed. The presence of a Romberg sign is defined as an increase in the patient's unsteadiness when the eyes are closed, whereas its absence is defined as no change when the eyes are open and then closed. The patient may be very unsteady; but if he is equally unsteady with eyes open compared to eyes closed, then the Romberg sign is absent. The maintenance of balance requires information as to the position of the body in space provided by the proprioceptive system (dorsal column, medial lemniscus), vestibular system, and visual cues. A normally functioning cerebellum is also necessary to assimilate this information and coordinate posture. If there is unsteadiness with the patient's eyes open, the cerebellum or its pathways are at fault. If unsteadiness worsens with the eyes closed, the proprioceptive and/or vestibular systems are implicated.

A Horner's syndrome (partial eyelid ptosis, pupillary miosis, and hemifacial anhidrosis) is produced by a lesion of the sympathetic pathway. The first-order neuron, which runs from the hypothalamus to the intermediolateral cell column of the C8 to T1 region of the spinal cord, runs through the dorsolateral tegmentum of the brainstem and is involved in this patient's lesion. Note that in this case the ptosis was incomplete compared to the complete ptosis secondary to an oculomotor nerve lesion described in case 3. The partial ptosis seen in Horner's syndrome is due to weakness of the tarsal muscle of Müller innervated by sympathetic nerves. The eyelid levator muscle is still intact and prevents the eyelid from drooping completely. A complete ptosis is usually indicative of an oculomotor nerve lesion.

The anatomic lesion is, therefore, located in the lateral medulla on the right side. The pathologic differential diagnosis of brainstem lesions includes (1) ischemic or hemorrhagic stroke, (2) trauma, (3) primary or metastatic tumors, (4) infection (e.g., abscess), (5) inflammatory processes, (6) demyelinating disease, and (7) degenerative disease. Since the onset was acute and there is no history of trauma, the neurologic differential diagnosis favors those processes related to cerebrovascular disease. The lateral medulla is perfused by a branch of the vertebral artery. Occlusion of the vertebral artery produces an infarct in the lateral medulla. Thrombosis of the right vertebral artery was seen on arteriography, confirming the neurologic diagnosis as an infarction of the right lateral medulla. The constellation of findings seen in this patient is called the lateral medullary or Wallenberg's syndrome.

**Case 6**

# Loss of Vision in the Right Eye, History of Right-Sided Weakness and Left-Sided Numbness

# Case 6

A 32-year-old woman was in her usual state of excellent health until one morning she noted that she could not see well enough out of her right eye to apply her make-up. She noted that she could see forms in the periphery of the visual field of her right eye but not when she looked directly at the object. Associated with the loss of vision was pain behind the right globe. The pain was made worse by eye movement. She could see perfectly well out of the left eye. There was no double vision.

Her previous medical history was remarkable for one episode 2 years earlier of dragging the right lower extremity while walking and experiencing difficulty ascending or descending stairs. She also recalled decreased ability to sense warm or cold water with the left leg when she took a bath. The lower-extremity symptoms improved over a few weeks.

Visual acuity was 20/200 with the right eye and 20/20 with the left eye. The patient's visual fields, shown in Figure 6-1A, are drawn so that one is seeing what the patient would see. (In visual field testing the visual threshold of each eye is tested independently with objects that vary in size and color or luminance. Areas of visual loss are denoted with darkened areas. The concentric lines represent visual thresholds to the different targets, with large bright targets seen normally in the far periphery when moved in toward the center and small dim targets only in the central field of vision.) The pupillary response to light was sluggish and incomplete when the light was directed into the right eye (Fig. 6-1B). However, for light directed into the left eye, both pupils constricted normally (Fig. 6-1B). When the light was swung from the left eye to the right eye, both pupils enlarged. Funduscopic examination was normal. There was slight weakness and increased tone in the right lower extremity. The right knee and right ankle tendon reflexes were hyperactive, whereas the other tendon reflexes were normal. A Babinski's sign on the right side was present. A slight decrease in pinprick sensation was noted in the left leg over the L2 through S2 dermatomes. The remainder of the neurologic examination was normal.

Consider first the abnormal pupillary light reflex on the right side. What anatomic structures and pathways mediate the pupillary light reflex?

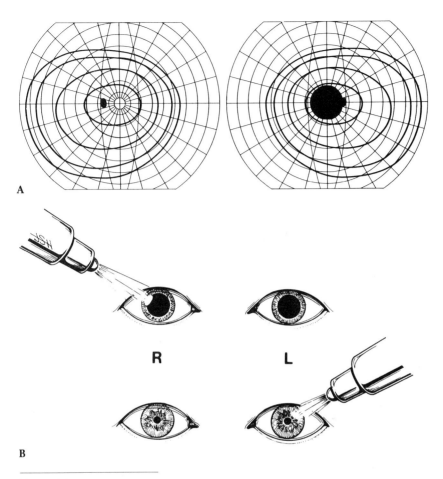

FIGURE 6-1.

The pathway for the pupillary light reflex (Fig. 6-2) begins in the retina. The axons from the retinal ganglion cell (RET) run through the optic nerve (ON), optic chiasm (CHI), and optic tract (OT) and—bypassing the lateral geniculate nucleus—synapse in the pretectal nucleus (PTN) of the midbrain at the level of the oculomotor nerve. Fibers then run from the pretectal nucleus to both Edinger-Westphal nuclei (EWN) of the oculomotor nerve nuclear complex. The nerve fibers from the EWN run in the oculomotor nerve to the ciliary ganglion (CG) and then through the short ciliary nerves to the iris sphincter. Therefore, when a light is directed into one eye, the information regarding light brightness is summated in the pretectal region of the midbrain and goes to both EWN equally. Consequently, both pupils constrict equally when a bright light is directed into one eye. If, for whatever cause (e.g., optic nerve lesion, retinal detachment, opacified cornea), less light brightness information is conducted through an optic nerve, less light is sensed in the pretectum of the midbrain. Both EWN receive less input, and the pupillary response is bilaterally sluggish or absent (directly and consensually) to the uniocular light stimulus to the involved eye. When the light is projected into the normal eye, both pupils then constrict briskly.

In this case, when a bright light was directed into the right eye, both pupils reacted sluggishly. When the light was swung over to the left eye, both pupils briskly constricted. Therefore, the efferent arc (oculomotor nerve) of the light reflex to the right eye was functioning normally, and the lesion must have been along the afferent limb of the reflex arc (optic nerve). Fibers carrying light brightness information cross at the optic chiasm. Since the patient had a uni-ocular rather than a hemianopic deficit, the lesion must have been anterior to the optic chiasm in the right optic nerve or retina. This relative afferent pupillary defect is also called the Marcus Gunn pupillary sign.

Other findings help to localize this lesion further. Since ocular and funduscopic examination did not reveal abnormalities of the cornea, lens, ocular media, or macula, the lesion had to be in the right optic nerve. Results of the "swinging flashlight test" for relative afferent pupillary defects supported this conclusion. In general, a macular lesion would cause only a slight relative afferent pupillary defect. Since the patient had a marked defect, this was further evidence that the lesion was in the right optic nerve.

Consider next the visual field loss. Where would the lesion most likely be to produce the patient's visual field deficit?

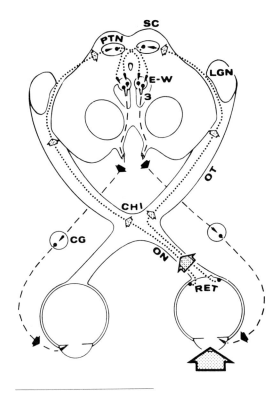

FIGURE 6-2.

3 = oculomotor (third nerve) nucleus; CG = ciliary ganglion; CHI = chiasm; E-W = Edinger-Westphal nucleus; LGN = lateral geniculate nucleus; ON = optic nerve; OT = optic tract; PTN = pretectal nucleus; RET = retina; SC = superior colliculus. Reproduced with permission from Glaser, J. *Neuro-ophthalmology.* Hagerstown, Md.: Harper & Row, 1978.

The pathway subserving the afferent visual system begins in the retinal ganglion cell and passes through the optic nerve. Fibers from the nasal half (medial to the fovea) of the retina cross to the opposite side in the optic chiasm, and those from the temporal (lateral) half remain uncrossed. Fibers then pass through the optic tract to synapse in the lateral geniculate nucleus of the thalamus. A second-order neuron leaves the lateral geniculate nucleus and passes through the optic radiations to reach the primary visual cortex in the occipital lobe. The fibers from the inferior retina (which convey visual information from the superior visual field) stay inferior throughout the visual system, run through the temporal lobe (Meyer's loop), and terminate in the inferior calcarine cortex. The fibers from the superior retina stay superior and course through the parietal lobe to end in the superior calcarine cortex (Fig. 6-3).

Lesions of the optic chiasm or lesions behind the optic chiasm cause defects in the visual fields of both eyes (i.e., bitemporal hemianopsia with chiasmal lesions, Fig. 6-3, lesion 2) and homonymous hemianopsia with retrochiasmal lesions (Fig. 6-3, lesion 8). It is important to note that a complete lesion of the visual pathway anywhere from the optic tract to the calcarine cortex will cause a total homonymous hemianopsia (Fig. 6-3, number 8). Less damaging lesions will give the partial homonymous hemianopsias seen in Figure 6-3, lesions 3 through 7, 9 through 11. Since the patient's visual defect is monocular, it must be prechiasmal (Fig. 6-3, lesion 1), consistent with the relative afferent pupillary defect due to a right optic nerve lesion.

The anatomy of the optic nerve and its surrounding structures determines the pathologic differential diagnosis. The common lesions of the optic nerve are (1) disorders of the myelin sheath (optic neuritis), (2) neoplasia of glia (optic nerve glioma), (3) neoplasia of the optic nerve sheath (optic nerve sheath meningioma), (4) ischemia of the optic nerve (ischemic optic neuropathy), and (5) optic nerve compression from disorders of other orbital contents (e.g., extraocular muscle enlargement in Graves' disease, metastatic tumors, and vascular tumors such as hemangiomas).

The neurologic differential diagnosis should account for the entire neurologic clinical presentation. Recall that the patient had an episode of right lower extremity weakness, hypertonia, hyperreflexia and Babinski's sign with decreased left lower extremity pinprick, and temperature sensation. Where is the lesion that would produce these findings? How does it relate to the patient's optic nerve findings?

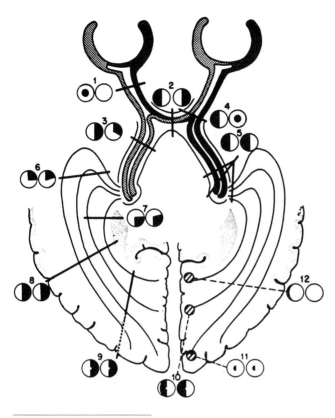

FIGURE 6-3.
Reproduced with permission from Harrington, D. O. *The Visual Fields* (5th ed.). St. Louis: Mosby, 1981.

The lower extremity findings of right-sided weakness with pinprick and temperature loss on the left side are findings of the Brown-Séquard syndrome (case 1) of the right half of the spinal cord. The lesion affects corticospinal fibers to the right lower extremity and fibers of the ascending right spinothalamic tract after they have crossed from the left side of the spinal cord (Fig. 6-4). If the dorsal columns are involved, there is also loss of vibratory sensation and proprioception on the ipsilateral side. This lesion, affecting lower but not upper extremities, must lie caudal to T1 and rostral to L2 levels of the cord. The pathologic differential diagnosis for the spinal cord lesion includes (1) disorders of the myelin sheath, (2) neoplasia, either primary or metastatic, (3) compression due to disease of the vertebral column, and (4) vascular disease, such as an arteriovascular malformation.

Thus, there are two separate sites in the anatomic diagnosis for this patient: right optic nerve and right spinal cord. Symptoms occurred at two separate times. It is most parsimonious to assume that both lesions were caused by the same process. Therefore, those items common to each pathologic differential diagnosis would constitute the neurologic differential diagnosis.

The most likely explanation (neurologic diagnosis) for these two lesions in a 32-year-old woman would be multiple sclerosis, which is a demyelinating disease that, by clinical definition, involves more than one CNS anatomic site. Demyelination in the optic nerve explains the visual findings, while demyelination in the spinal cord explains the patient's lower extremity weakness and sensory loss.

The diagnosis of multiple sclerosis is often difficult, since the plaques of demyelination are multifocal. Multiple sclerosis can present in a variety of ways and is usually characterized by episodic exacerbations and remissions. There is no one specific symptom or symptom complex or laboratory test that is pathognomonic for this disorder. The diagnosis requires evidence of multiple CNS anatomic sites of lesions, exacerbations and remissions, involvement of white matter, and exclusion of other likely diagnoses.

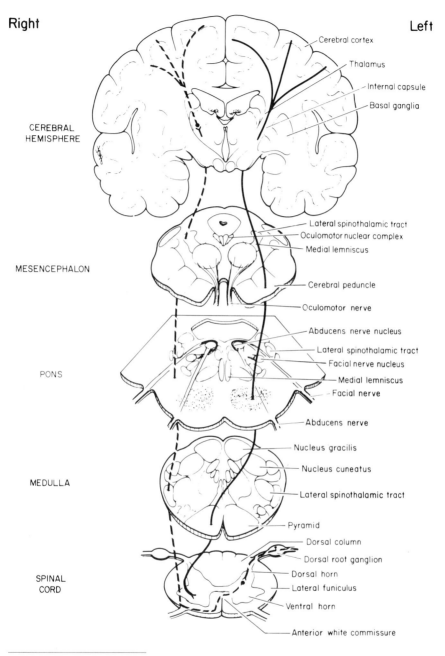

FIGURE 6-4.
Solid line: corticospinal tract; dashed line: lateral spinothalamic tract.

**Case 7**

# Left-Sided Weakness, Left Gaze Paresis, and Left Visual Field Loss

*Right middle Cerebral Infarction: See table*

# Case 7

While eating breakfast, a 59-year-old right-handed man with hypertension and diabetes mellitus dropped a glass of juice that he had been holding in his left hand. His speech became slurred, and he noted numbness over the left half of his body. He was able to walk, but he dragged his left foot. His wife, noting no change in his condition over several hours, brought him to the hospital.

His vital signs were normal except for an irregular pulse. He was alert and oriented. His speech was slurred but otherwise fluent, and comprehension was normal. His gaze was consistently directed toward his right, and he was unable to bring his eyes past the midline when asked to look to the left. When he was asked to look at the examiner, who then passively rotated his head in the horizontal plane, his eyes moved conjugately and fully (i.e., his gaze paresis could be overcome by the doll's-head, or oculocephalic, maneuver). His visual field defect is shown in Figure 7-1. The muscles of facial expression in the lower portion of the left face were moderately weak, and there was moderate weakness of the left arm and mild weakness of the left leg. On the left side, the tendon reflexes were hyperactive and Babinski's sign was present. Light touch, pinprick, and warm and cold stimuli were accurately identified over the face and limbs. With his eyes closed, however, he was imprecise in localizing where on his left limbs a particular stimulus was applied. Proprioceptive sensation was impaired on the left side. With his eyes closed, he was unable to identify coins placed in his left hand (astereognosis) or to name figures traced in the palm of his left hand (agraphesthesia). With his eyes closed, he was able to identify which of his hands was individually touched by the examiner. However, when both hands were touched simultaneously, he stated that only the right side was touched (left-sided extinction to double simultaneous stimulation).

Consider the patient's left-sided weakness and sensory findings. What functional systems are involved?

---

*Handwritten notes:*

Motor      Sensory

↓ Left hand + foot

↓ Slurred speech   — ok Comprehension Normal

↓ gaze directed Rt
couldn't bring eyes past midline
Normal VOR

↓ Left face muscles (Lower face)

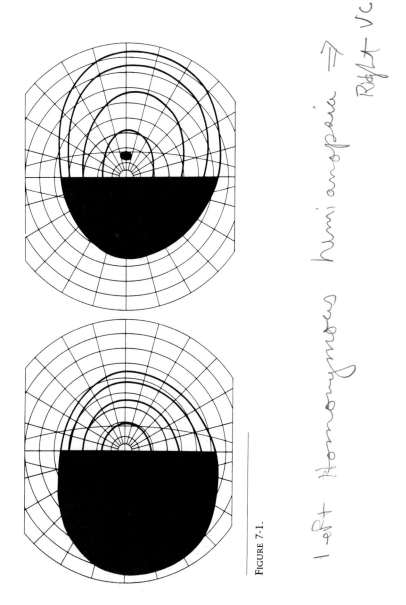

FIGURE 7-1.

1 Left Homonymous hemianopsia → Right VC

Case 7

U.MN. { The symptoms of dragging the left leg and inability to grasp with left hand and signs of left-sided weakness, hyperreflexia, and Babinski's sign are evidence of an upper motoneuron lesion. Since the arm and leg are involved, a lesion of the corticospinal tract must be present at or above the C4 level of the spinal cord (solid line, Fig. 7-2). Involvement of the lower portion of the left side of the face implies an upper motoneuron lesion above the level of the facial nuclei (solid-dot-solid line, Fig. 7-2) (see case 2). Therefore, the patient's motor system lesion is rostral to the lower pons (Fig. 7-2).

Somesthetic sensation is primarily carried in two major systems: the spinothalamic and the medial lemniscal. The spinothalamic system mediates pain and temperature sensation (Fig. 7-2, dashed line). The first-order neuron has its cell body in the dorsal root ganglion. Its axons enter the spinal cord and synapse on the second-order neurons. The second-order neuron axons ascend one or two segments, cross near the region of the central canal, ascend in the contralateral spinothalamic tract of the lateral funiculus, and synapse on the third-order neurons in the ventral posterior lateral nucleus of the thalamus. The third-order neuron leaves the thalamus, ascends in the posterior limb of the internal capsule and the corona radiata, and terminates in the somatosensory cortex of the postcentral gyrus (Brodmann's cortical areas 3, 1, and 2).

The other major somatosensory system, the medial lemniscus system, mediates such sensations as graphesthesia, vibration, and proprioception. The first-order neuron of this system also lies in the dorsal root ganglion. Its axon enters the spinal cord and ascends ipsilaterally (Fig. 7-2, dotted line) to synapse on the second-order neuron cell bodies of the nuclei cuneatus and gracilis. The axons of the second-order neurons cross to the other side, enter the medial lemniscus, and ascend to the third-order neurons in the ventral posterior lateral nucleus of the thalamus. These third-order neurons project to the somatosensory cortex in the parietal lobe.

Patients with lesions of the somatosensory cortex that spare the thalamus continue to appreciate touch, pain, and temperature stimuli (elementary sensory modalities) but may be unable to localize precisely the area being stimulated. The discriminative or cortical sensations (proprioception, stereognosis, graphesthesia, two-point discrimination, the ability to localize light touch) require a normally functioning cerebral cortex as well as medial lemniscus system. Since the patient had intact primary modalities but loss of cortical modalities on the left side, his lesion had to be rostral to the right thalamus. Therefore, the patient has a lesion of the right hemisphere involving the corticospinal and somatosensory functional systems.

Are the patient's visual deficits consistent with this localization? How can one explain the patient's left gaze palsy?

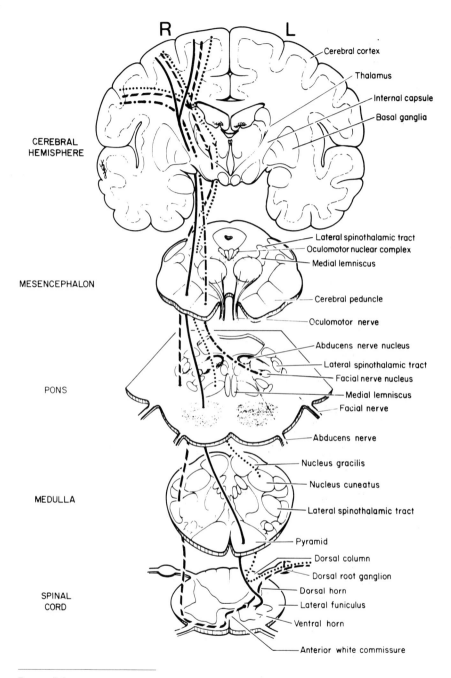

FIGURE 7-2.
Solid line: corticospinal tract; dashed line: lateral spinothalamic tract; dotted line: medial lemniscal system; solid-dot-solid line: corticobulbar fibers to facial nerve nucleus.

The pathway for the control of horizontal gaze begins in the frontal eye fields (Brodmann's area 8), an area of the cerebral cortex just anterior to the motor facial representation of the precentral gyrus. The pathway (frontopontine tract) descends through the cerebral white matter and internal capsule and crosses in the lower midbrain to reach the paramedian pontine reticular formation on the contralateral side (Fig. 7-3). Stimulation of the paramedian pontine reticular formation causes the eyes to deviate conjugately to the ipsilateral side, whereas destructive lesions cause the eyes to deviate contralaterally. Therefore, a lesion above the lower midbrain of pathways from the right frontal eye fields will prevent the patient from looking to the contralateral side.

In the presented case, the eyes are conjugately deviated to the right, and the patient cannot voluntarily look conjugately to the left. Involvement of the left paramedian pontine reticular formation or the frontopontine tract below the lower midbrain would be inconsistent with the patient's left hemiparesis, because the involved corticospinal tract runs on the right side of the pons. However, a right-sided lesion above the lower midbrain affecting the frontal eye fields or their descending fibers and the corticospinal fibers would produce the patient's left gaze paresis and the left-sided weakness.

Although the patient was unable to look voluntarily to the left, his eyes could be brought to the left with a doll's-head or oculocephalic maneuver; that is, when the patient fixated on a target and his head was briskly turned in the horizontal plane, the eyes moved fully relative to the head. This movement requires a normally functioning oculovestibular eye movement system, which produces eye movements of equal magnitude to, but in the opposite direction of, any head movement, thus enabling the patient to keep a target in focus on the fovea when the head moves.

The pathway for this oculovestibular eye movement begins in the semicircular canals. Here, sensory neurons send axons via the vestibulocochlear nerve to synapse in the vestibular nuclei. For horizontal gaze, the vestibular nuclei project to the abducens nucleus in the brainstem and through the medial longitudinal fasciculus to the oculomotor and trochlear nuclei. If a gaze paresis can be overcome by using the oculovestibular eye movement system, as in this patient, it implies that oculomotor, trochlear, abducens nuclei and nerves, and medial longitudinal fasciculus are intact, and the lesion must be above their level. Loss of volitional eye movements with preservation of oculovestibular eye movements is called a supranuclear disorder of gaze.

**W**hat is the patient's visual field defect, and where must a lesion be to produce it? Is the presumptive anatomic localization of a lesion involving the frontal eye fields consistent with the field defect?

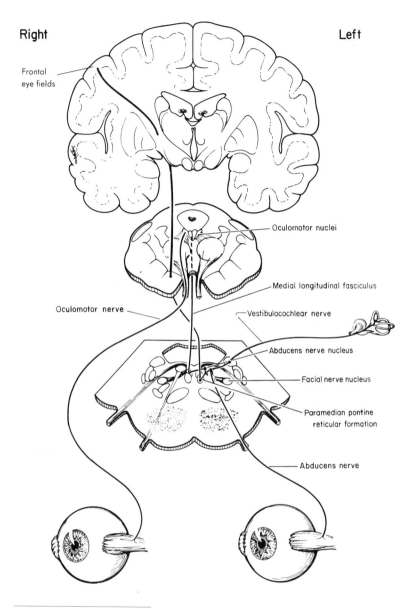

FIGURE 7-3.
Solid line: frontopontine tract.

A left homonymous hemianopsia follows right-sided lesions of the retrochiasmal afferent visual system, including the optic tract, lateral geniculate nucleus, optic radiations, and occipital cortex (Fig. 7-4). The optic radiations course just posterior to the major somatosensory area in the parietal lobe. Therefore, if one extends the lesion of the right hemisphere from the frontal eye fields, motor cortex, and sensory cortex to the optic radiations, the anatomic diagnosis is complete.

The list of possibilities in the pathologic differential diagnosis is long. What are the relevant possibilities that constitute the neurologic differential diagnosis?

The onset of symptoms was abrupt, which suggests either a vascular or electrical (seizure) cause. Brain tumors usually produce gradual neurologic deficits. (Caution is required, however; infrequently, brain tumors may present abruptly, either by causing seizures or by affecting the circulation through vascular compression or erosion or by shunting blood away). Seizures usually produce such "positive" (excessive function) symptoms as paresthesia, visual hallucinations, and tonic-clonic motor activity. These were not present in this case. Seizures rarely produce purely negative symptoms (loss of function). Therefore, a vascular cause is more likely. However, hemorrhages are often accompanied by signs—not present in this case—of meningeal irritation or increased intracranial pressure. The more likely vascular mechanism is occlusion.

The blood vessels supplying the brain have specific anatomic distributions. If the symptoms and signs of this case are due to a lesion of an artery supplying the brain, then the anatomic localization must be consistent with the territory of the brain supplied by that artery. Is the anatomic localization deduced in this case so consistent?

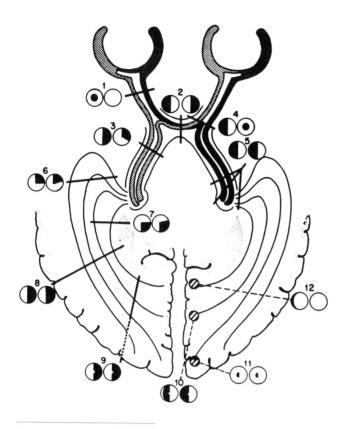

FIGURE 7-4.

1 = optic nerve—central scotoma on side of lesion, with normal contralateral field; 2 = chiasm—bitemporal hemianopsia; 3 = optic tract—contralateral incongruous homonymous hemianopsia; 4 = optic nerve—chiasmal junction; central scotoma on side of lesion with contralateral temporal hemianopsia or hemianopic scotoma; 5 = posterior optic tract, external geniculate ganglion, posterior limb of internal capsule—complete contralateral homonymous hemianopsia or incomplete incongruous contralateral homonymous hemianopsia; 6 = optic radiation; anterior loop in temporal lobe—incongruous contralateral homonymous hemianopsia or superior quadrantanopsia; 7 = medial fibers of optic radiation—contralateral incongruous inferior homonymous quadrantanopsia; 8 = optic radiation in parietal lobe—contralateral homonymous hemianopsia, sometimes slightly incongruous, with minimal macular sparing; 9 = optic radiation in posterior parietal lobe and occipital lobe—contralateral congruous, homonymous hemianopsia with macular sparing; 10 = midportion of calcarine cortex—contralateral congruous homonymous hemianopsia with wide macular sparing and sparing of contralateral temporal crescent; 11 = tip of occipital lobe—contralateral congruous homonymous hemianoptic scotomas; 12 = anterior tip of calcarine fissure—contralateral loss of temporal crescent with otherwise normal visual fields. Reproduced with permission from Harrington, D. O. *The Visual Fields* (5th ed.). St. Louis: Mosby, 1981.

Figure 7-5 shows the regions of the brain supplied by the major arteries. The arterial system is divided into two divisions. The first is the anterior circulation supplied by the internal carotid artery. The internal carotid artery divides into the ophthalmic artery, anterior cerebral artery, middle cerebral artery, and posterior communicating artery. The last links the anterior circulation to the second division, the posterior circulation. The posterior circulation is made up of the vertebral arteries, which give off the posterior inferior cerebellar arteries and then join to form the basilar artery. The basilar artery then gives off several branches before finally dividing to form the posterior cerebral arteries. (Some of the major signs and symptoms caused by disease in the anterior or posterior circulations are listed in Table 7-1.)

The anterior cerebral arteries supply the frontal and medial aspects of the cerebrum (Fig. 7-5). In this distribution is the area of the motor and sensory cortex that represents the lower extremities. Strokes in this distribution would be expected to produce contralateral lower extremity weakness and sensory loss. The posterior cerebral artery supplies the occipital (visual) cortex, upper brainstem, and inferior temporal lobe. Lesions of this vessel do not affect the motor or sensory cortex, as in the present case, but often produce loss of vision in the contralateral visual field. The middle cerebral artery supplies most of the lateral aspect of the cerebrum, including most of the motor and sensory cortices and frontal eye fields. In addition, the middle cerebral artery also supplies much of the underlying white matter, such as the optic radiations. Therefore, a stroke in the distribution of the middle cerebral artery produces contralateral weakness, sensory loss, homonymous hemianopsia, and loss of voluntary gaze to the contralateral side. In this case, it is clear that a stroke in the distribution of the middle cerebral artery is consistent with the anatomic diagnosis and is the first item in the present neurologic differential diagnosis.

The patient has hypertension and diabetes mellitus, significant risk factors for developing atherosclerotic disease. Atherosclerosis has a predilection for specific anatomic sites. In disease of the anterior circulation, the carotid artery bifurcation, a site of hemodynamic turbulence, is the most common site of atherosclerotic lesions. It is important to remember that there are many causes of stroke other than atherosclerosis (e.g., cardiac emboli, polycythemia vera, thrombocytosis). Recall that this patient's pulse was irregular. Further evaluation revealed that he had atrial fibrillation, and the cause of his stroke was an embolus from his left atrium to his right middle cerebral artery.

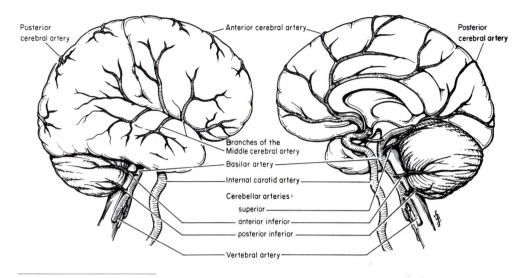

FIGURE 7-5.

Table 7-1.
Common symptoms and signs of ischemia or infarct relative to circulation affected

| Anterior Circulation | Posterior Circulation |
|---|---|
| Contralateral to lesion<br>  Weakness of face, arm, and leg<br>  Numbness of face, arm, and leg<br>  Homonymous hemianopsia<br>  Supranuclear horizontal conjugate gaze paresis<br>Aphasia (left cerebral hemisphere in right-handers)<br>Neglect syndrome (right cerebral hemisphere in right-handers) | Loss of consciousness<br>Quadriparesis or hemiparesis<br>Blindness or homonymous hemianopsia<br>Vertigo<br>Diplopia<br>Dysarthria<br>Dysphagia<br>Ataxia<br>Hoarseness<br>Gaze paresis (horizontal or vertical, supranuclear, nuclear, or internuclear)<br>Paresis of oculomotor, trochlear, and abducens nerves |

# Case 8

# Galactorrhea and Double Vision

## Case 8

A 31-year-old woman had experienced double vision for the previous 2 weeks. She said that one image was off to one side and higher than the other image. She also noticed that her left eyelid had been drooping for the previous week. On further questioning, she stated that since the birth of her last child 3 years earlier she had not had a menstrual period. She breast-fed her last child for only 2 months but continued to have a daily milky discharge from her breasts. Mild bifrontal head pain had been present intermittently for 6 months.

Milk was expressible from her breasts (galactorrhea). Visual acuity was 20/20 bilaterally. With confrontation visual field testing she was unable to see fingers in the superior temporal field of either eye. Testing of the visual field by formal perimetry showed the visual field defects pictured in Figure 8-1. When she was asked to look straight ahead, her left eye was deviated down and to the left, and her left palpebral fissure was 3 mm narrower than the right. The left pupil measured 5 mm in diameter and the right pupil was 2 mm. The left pupil reacted sluggishly when light was directed into either eye and also when she looked at a near target. The pupillary light reflex in the right eye was normal. She was able to abduct the eye normally but could not adduct, elevate, or depress the left globe. She was able to detect mild fragrances with either nostril. Sensation to light touch and pinprick in all three divisions of the fifth cranial nerve was normal, as were the corneal reflexes. The remainder of the cranial nerve examination was normal. Motor, sensory, tendon reflex, coordination, and gait examinations were also normal.

Involvement of which cranial nerve(s) accounts for the patient's ocular motility disturbance?

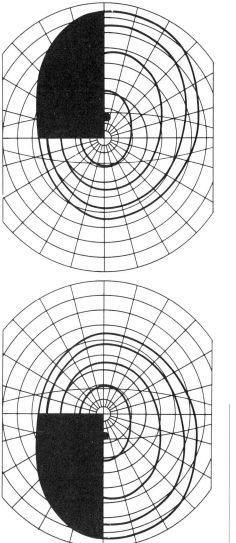

FIGURE 8-1.

Case 8

The functions of the oculomotor (third cranial) nerve are elevation, depression, and adduction of the globe. This cranial nerve also innervates the levator muscle of the eyelid and carries parasympathetic fibers to the iris sphincter. The functions of the trochlear (fourth cranial) nerve are intorsion, depression, and slight abduction. The abducens (sixth cranial) nerve abducts the eye. The patient, therefore, had a lesion of the oculomotor nucleus or nerve.

The nucleus of the oculomotor nerve lies in the mesencephalon (Fig. 8-2). Fibers from the superior rectus subnucleus of the oculomotor nucleus cross through the oculomotor nucleus to innervate the contralateral superior rectus muscle. On the other hand, subnuclei for the medial rectus, inferior oblique, and inferior rectus innervate muscles ipsilateral to their origin. The nuclei for the levator muscles of the eyelids lie in the midline, as do the paired midline Edinger-Westphal nuclei, which innervate the iris sphincter. Therefore, a unilateral midbrain lesion involving the oculomotor nerve nucleus would also usually involve both the Edinger-Westphal nuclei and levator nuclei along with the nuclei for the extraocular muscles, producing bilateral ptosis, bilateral dilated unreactive pupils, and bilateral loss of upgaze along with paresis of adduction and depression of the eye on the side of the lesion. The lesion in this case was of the nerve after it leaves the nucleus, because in the contralateral eye there was no ptosis, pupillary dilatation, or elevation deficit. Therefore, the lesion had to be along the course of the nerve between the nucleus and the orbit. Since the third nerve passes through the cerebral peduncles and the patient did not have a hemiparesis, the lesion had to be outside the midbrain.

After the oculomotor nerve exits the midbrain, it passes between the posterior cerebral and superior cerebellar arteries. The nerve then courses near the free edge of the tentorium and the posterior communicating artery and enters the cavernous sinus. In the anterior portion of the cavernous sinus, the nerve divides into a superior division, which innervates the levator palpebrae superioris and the superior rectus muscles, and an inferior division, which innervates the pupil, medial rectus, inferior rectus, and inferior oblique muscles.

**M**ore information is needed to refine the anatomic diagnosis. Where must the lesion be in the afferent visual system to produce this visual field defect?

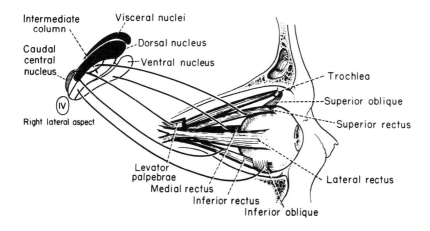

FIGURE 8-2.
Reproduced with permission from Carpenter, M. B. *Human Neuroanatomy* (7th ed.). Baltimore: Williams & Wilkins, 1976.

Although the patient revealed no visual symptoms, she had a superior bitemporal quadrantanopsia. The temporal visual field projects onto the nasal retina, whose fibers enter the optic nerve and cross in the optic chiasm (Fig. 8-3A). Therefore, in order to have a bitemporal hemianopic field defect, there must be a lesion of the optic chiasm. This implies that the oculomotor nerve is affected near the optic chiasm, if one is to explain the patient's deficit by a single lesion.

What is the pathologic differential diagnosis of lesions of the optic chiasm? Knowing the anatomy of the structures related to the optic chiasm helps (Fig. 8-3B). Understanding the types of diseases that might affect that anatomy allow one to formulate a differential diagnosis.

The pituitary gland lies just below the chiasm. Expansion of pituitary tumors above the confines of the sella turcica may compress the optic chiasm from below. Meningiomas of the tuberculum sella can also compress the optic chiasm to cause bitemporal hemianopsia. The internal carotid and the anterior communicating arteries are adjacent to the optic chiasm, and aneurysms of these vessels can also compress the chiasm. The frontal and temporal lobes border the chiasm, and tumors or abscesses of this region can thus affect the chiasm. Remnants of the embryologic Rathke's pouch lying in the midline above and below the optic chiasm can give rise to tumors (craniopharyngiomas), causing bitemporal hemianopsias.

Was the optic chiasm being compressed from above or below? Remember that fibers from the inferior retina subserving the superior visual fields stay inferior throughout the afferent visual system. Therefore, when the chiasm is compressed from below, the initial visual field abnormality will be a superior bitemporal quadrantanopsia. Thus, the pathologic differential diagnosis includes pituitary tumors, craniopharyngioma, aneurysms, dysgerminomas, and granulomatous disease (e.g., sarcoid, tuberculous). The patient's amenorrhea and galactorrhea imply that the lesion had also affected the endocrine system. Thus, the leading possibility in the neurologic differential diagnosis was a pituitary adenoma secreting prolactin.

Skull x-rays in this patient showed an enlarged sella turcica. A CT scan revealed a mass projecting up from the pituitary fossa. Arteriography showed no aneurysm. The patient underwent a transphenoidal resection of the mass, which was confirmed to be a prolactinoma.

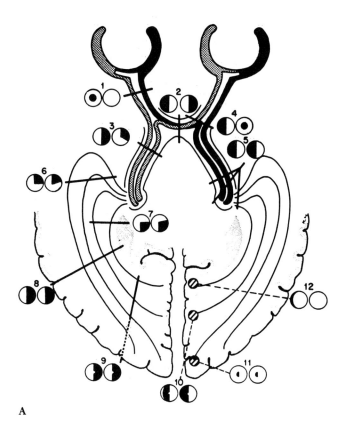

A

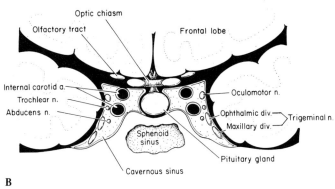

B

FIGURE 8-3.
See Fig. 7-4 (p. 87) for key to abbreviations. Fig. 8-3A reproduced with permission from Harrington, D. O. *The Visual Fields* (5th ed.). St. Louis: Mosby, 1981.

# Case 9

# Visual Loss with Olfactory Hallucinations and Altered Behavior

# Case 9

A 32-year-old computer programmer with a 4-month history of headaches sought medical advice because of a "strange spell." He had suddenly noticed a foul odor, described as something like burnt rubber. Fifteen seconds later a co-worker had noticed a motionless stare, which lasted 10 seconds. He then engaged in chewing, lip-smacking, grimacing, and swallowing movements, which lasted about 30 seconds. This was followed by a state of confusion, during which the patient arose from his desk, drank from the water fountain, returned to the desk, and began staring at his computer keyboard. Finally, he asked over and over, "Where is it?" His responses to his co-worker's questions seemed confused, but a few brief responses were appropriate. Over the next 5 minutes he gradually returned to normal. The patient recalled nothing of this episode other than the unexpected disagreeable odor. Three weeks earlier, while driving home, he had found himself sitting in his car on the side of the road in a neighboring town, uncertain where he was or how he had gotten there.

He was awake, alert, and attentive when examined. His mental status examination was normal. Cranial nerve examination was normal except for a visual field abnormality (Fig. 9-1). He correctly identified mild fragrances in each nostril. Pinprick, proprioceptive, and vibratory sensation was normal, as were strength, muscle tone, tendon reflexes, and rapid alternating movements. Finger-to-nose and heel-to-shin tasks were performed without ataxia or tremor, and gait was normal. The Romberg and Babinski signs were absent.

What anatomic systems are involved in producing the patient's olfactory hallucination and subsequent behavior?

To this point negative symptoms and signs have been the focus of attention. Positive symptoms and signs may also occur. The patient's symptom of a foul smell represents a positive symptom, whereas anosmia (inability to smell) would represent a negative symptom. Similarly, the chewing, lip-smacking, grimacing, and swallowing movements are positive symptoms. Seizures often produce positive symptoms, and their character reflects the underlying function of the part of the brain involved in the seizure. For example, a seizure arising from the motor cortex would produce involuntary jerking of the contralateral extremities.

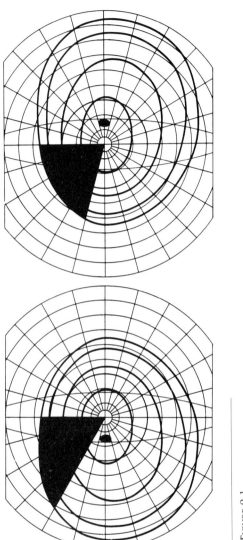

FIGURE 9-1.

The patient's olfactory hallucinations imply that the seizure discharge probably arose in the olfactory system. The pathways mediating smell begin in the olfactory sensory epithelium of the upper nasal cavity. Nerve fibers pierce the cribriform plate and enter the cranium to form the olfactory bulb. Fibers leave the bulb and course in the olfactory tract before dividing into the lateral and medial olfactory stria. Neurons are then distributed to the anterior olfactory nucleus, olfactory tubercle, amygdaloid and septal nuclei, and other structures in the deep medial frontal and temporal lobes (Fig. 9-2).

The patient had partial complex seizures. These seizures begin abruptly and usually last less than a minute. The aura, which represents the initial focal onset of the epileptic attack, can later be recalled by the patient. Symptoms may be visceral (e.g., ill-defined epigastric sensation, dizziness, salivation), perceptual (e.g., dèjá vu, jamais vu, visual illusions, hallucinations of smell or taste), emotional (e.g., fear, depression, anger), or cognitive (e.g., stereotyped words or thoughts, confusion). Stereotyped or reactive automatisms, for which the patient is amnestic, may follow. Stereotyped automatisms include repetitive semipurposeful movements, chewing, grimacing, lip smacking, or picking at one's clothes. Reactive automatisms are complex coordinated automatic behaviors that appear to be purposeful, e.g., repetitively washing one's hands. Such seizures were once thought to originate exclusively in the temporal lobe—hence the old term temporal lobe seizures. However, abnormal electrical discharges from other foci, such as the orbital frontal cortex, also cause partial complex seizures.

Further information is necessary to refine the anatomic diagnosis. Where must the lesion be to produce the patient's visual field loss?

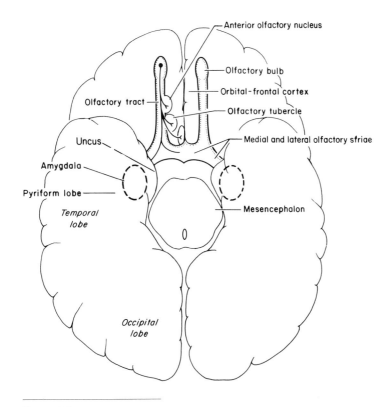

FIGURE 9-2.

As discussed in case 6, the pathway of the afferent visual system begins with the retinal ganglion cell and courses through the optic nerve. Fibers from the nasal retina cross in the optic chiasm and, with temporal retinal fibers from the other eye, synapse on the second-order neurons in the lateral geniculate nucleus. Axons of second-order neurons for the inferior visual field (superior retina) run through the parietal lobe to the superior bank of the calcarine sulcus of the occipital lobe. The fibers for the superior visual fields (from the inferior retina) go through the temporal lobe to reach the inferior bank of the calcarine sulcus.

The most posterior lesions of the visual system have the most congruous field defects (i.e., visual field plots for each eye appear more nearly identical). Compare lesion 6 with lesion 9 in Figure 9-3. Optic tract lesions are characteristically incongruous; lesions of the temporal and parietal lobes produce semicongruous visual field defects, and lesions of the occipital lobe cause exquisitely congruous homonymous defects. Therefore, this patient has a semicongruous left homonymous superior quadrantanopsia, which implies a right temporal lobe anatomic diagnosis (Fig. 9-3).

A routine electroencephalogram (EEG) showed nonspecific right temporal slowing, but an EEG with nasopharyngeal electrodes during sleep showed spikes in the right nasopharyngeal electrode. These electrodes abut against the posterior nasopharyngeal wall, are proximate to the orbital frontal cortex and medial temporal lobe, and may demonstrate electrical abnormalities not detected by more distant scalp electrodes.

The patient's history, physical examination, and EEG findings are consistent with a lesion of the right temporal lobe, which is the anatomic diagnosis. The pathologic differential diagnosis of lesions that affect the temporal lobe includes (1) ischemia or hemorrhage, (2) primary or metastatic tumors, (3) abscesses, (4) inflammatory disease, and (5) trauma. The 4-month history of headache is most consistent with an expanding mass lesion, and tumors (which are more common than abscesses) are the first items in the neurologic differential diagnosis. A CT scan showed a low-density, contrast-enhancing right temporal lobe lesion with some calcification present in the lesion. The mass was biopsied, and the neurologic diagnosis was found to be an oligodendroglioma.

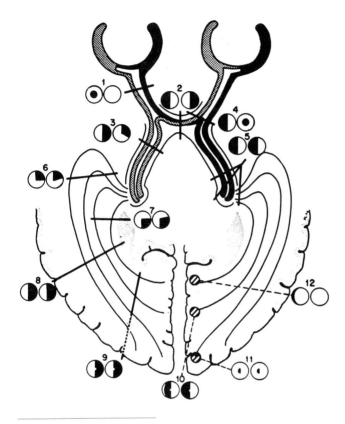

FIGURE 9-3.
1 = optic nerve—central scotoma on side of lesion, with normal contralateral field; 2 = chiasm—bitemporal hemianopsia; 3 = optic tract—contralateral incongruous homonymous hemianopsia; 4 = optic nerve—chiasmal junction; central scotoma on side of lesion with contralateral temporal hemianopsia or hemianopic scotoma; 5 = posterior optic tract, external geniculate ganglion, posterior limb of internal capsule—complete contralateral homonymous hemianopsia or incomplete incongruous contralateral homonymous hemianopsia; 6 = optic radiation; anterior loop in temporal lobe—incongruous contralateral hemianopsia or superior quadrantanopsia; 7 = medial fibers of optic radiation—contralateral incongruous inferior homonymous quadrantanopsia; 8 = optic radiation in parietal lobe—contralateral homonymous hemianopsia, sometimes slightly incongruous, with minimal macular sparing; 9 = optic radiation in posterior parietal lobe and occipital lobe—contralateral congruous, homonymous hemianopsia with macular sparing; 10 = midportion of calcarine cortex—contralateral congruous homonymous hemianopsia with wide macular sparing and sparing of contralateral temporal crescent; 11 = tip of occipital lobe—contralateral congruous homonymous hemianoptic scotomas; 12 = anterior tip of calcarine fissure—contralateral loss of temporal crescent with otherwise normal visual fields. Reproduced with permission from Harrington, D. O. *The Visual Fields* (5th ed.). St. Louis: Mosby, 1981.

**Case 10**

## Sudden Difficulty Speaking

*Conduction Problem*

*[Handwritten margin notes:*
- *difficulty speech (i.e. word finding prob./paraphasic errors)*
- *Comprehension Normal*
- *No other Sensory problems noted*
- *Cranial N Normal*
- *Paraphasic errors*
- *Naming errors*
- *repetition impair.*
- *Compreh. Normal]*

## Case 10

A 57-year-old right-handed man was hospitalized after an acute myocardial infarction. The day after his discharge, he was readmitted after suddenly developing difficulty speaking. Although he understood the speech of others, he was frustrated by his own mistakes in trying to speak. His wife explained, "The words just come out wrong." He denied changes in vision, strength, sensation, or gait.

He was alert and oriented. Cranial nerve functions, strength, coordination, tendon reflexes and gait were normal. He spoke clearly at a normal rate, using complete sentences. Frequently, however, he seemed unable to find the appropriate word, and some of his expressions were overly vague. He stumbled over some words and also made paraphasic errors (a paraphasia is the incorrect substitution of a similar-sounding word—as "giss" for kiss—or of a word similar in meaning—as "hug" for kiss). He also groped for the correct word and made paraphasic errors when he attempted to name items shown to him. Examples of these responses were "Uh, uh coat; no, a sleeve" (sleeve); and "that thing at the bottom of the sheeve, shreeve, sleeve; the caff, cuff" (cuff). Repetition of words and sentences spoken by the examiner was particularly impaired. Pencil was repeated as "prensle, pren, pencil"; one-quarter as "one-fourth"; fifty-seven as "forty-four"; shut the door as "close the blor...boar...door"; and no ifs, ands, or buts as "no bits, no bins, and buts." In contrast to his own communication difficulty, his comprehension of others' speech was normal. Errors in reading aloud resembled those of his spontaneous speech, but he fully understood what he read.

An anatomic diagnosis for the so-called higher cerebral functions is approached in the same manner as that for impairments like weakness or decreased sensation. For example, language functions are to a large extent organized anatomically, and lesions in different brain regions impair language differently. Symptoms and signs resulting from lesions of these systems can be localized using the same logical approach employed with earlier cases.

Decide how the patient's communication is affected. Is the impairment one of dysarthria, aphasia, or both? What functional system is involved?

Acquired defects in speaking assume two general forms: impaired articulation (dysarthria) and impaired language (aphasia). Dysarthria is limited to the spoken word; aphasia almost always includes defects in both oral and written language. The dysarthric patient understands perfectly the speech of others, but many aphasics are impaired in both speech production and comprehension. Dysarthria is best considered as a special sign of damage to motor (or occasionally sensory) systems, whereas aphasia follows lesions within a functional language system.

Common to all aphasic syndromes is an inability to provide or use words correctly (word-finding difficulty). At times this is the only disturbance (anomic aphasia), but word-finding difficulty may also be overshadowed by other, more glaring, language deficits. Whenever aphasia is suspected, the examiner must assess the patient's ability to name objects in his spontaneous speech and, more formally, to provide names for specific items. In practice, one presents test objects visually (visual confrontation naming), asking the patient for the proper name.

Language deficits of aphasia are not confined to a single sensory modality. Thus, the aphasic who has difficulty naming a key on a visual confrontation task would have comparable difficulty in naming a key when blindfolded and asked to identify it by palpation or by listening to the jangle of a bunch of keys. Patients unable to name items presented visually but who are nonetheless successful for items presented in other modalities have either a visual perceptual deficit or, much more uncommonly, a lesion that precludes certain visual information from reaching regions of the brain important for language functions.

Though he made paraphasic errors (such as "bloor" for door and "forty-four" for fifty-seven), the patient's speech was enunciated clearly. His defect was solely one of the language system, that is, a linguistic disturbance in the production or comprehension of words used in communication. Emotional overtones of speech, though properly considered a form of communication, are excluded in this definition of language. Brain lesions that impair the production and recognition of affective information occur outside traditional language areas. Such lesions are often in the right cerebral hemisphere. In right-handed persons, aphasia almost always implies left cerebral hemisphere injury. For left-handers the converse is not necessarily true. Although more than half of left-handers are also left hemisphere language-dominant, some have right hemisphere or bilateral language representation. For right-handers lesions in left hemisphere subcortical structures, such as the thalamus and putamen, occasionally disturb language, but the usual site of damage of aphasia is predominantly cortical. One can thus conclude that the patient probably has cortical damage of the left hemisphere.

The next step is to localize further this left-sided cortical lesion. Anomia alone would imply only that there is dysfunction somewhere within the left hemisphere language system. However, the presence of other language disturbances permits a more specific anatomic diagnosis within this functional system.

Two cortical regions adjacent to the left sylvian fissure are particularly important within the language system. The more anterior of these perisylvian language centers, Broca's area, includes the posterior part of the left inferior (third) frontal gyrus. It is immediately in front of the premotor area concerned with movements of the lips, tongue, pharynx, and larynx. A posterior center, Wernicke's area, includes the posterior portion of the superior (first) temporal gyrus behind the primary auditory cortex of the left hemisphere. Broca's area, Wernicke's area, and pathways connecting the two (probably the white matter bundle known as the arcuate fasciculus) form the perisylvian core of the language system. It thus includes inferior portions of the left frontal and parietal lobes and the superior portion of the left temporal lobe.

Consider the patient's inability to repeat phrases spoken by the examiner. What does this impairment imply as to the lesion producing his aphasia?

In a simplified overview of brain function, frontal or anterior cortical regions are concerned with motor programming, and more posterior regions with sensory perception. Similarly, language regions behind the central sulcus are more involved with speech reception and comprehension, and frontal regions are more concerned with speech production. A left hemisphere transcortical zone surrounding the language core has important but anatomically ill-defined connections with the adjacent core. Transcortical lesions result in language deficits similar to but usually less severe than those caused by damage to the perisylvian areas. Because connections between Wernicke's and Broca's areas are intact, transcortical aphasics are able to repeat phrases and sentences, whereas patients with perisylvian lesions cannot. The auditory cortex of the superior temporal lobes is necessary for the perception of all sound, including speech. Rare patients with bilateral injury to these areas may be "cortically deaf."

Wernicke's area is a higher-order auditory association area involved in the comprehension of linguistically important sounds (speech). It may also be important for understanding language in nonauditory modalities, such as written language (reading). For repetition to occur, connections between Wernicke's and Broca's area must also be intact. The requisite linking pathway is probably the arcuate fasciculus. Finally, Broca's area and the adjacent motor cortex are required for the reproduction of speech originally perceived in the temporal lobe. Because the patient's repetition is impaired, his anatomic diagnosis must include left hemisphere regions near the sylvian fissure, the perisylvian language core. (Fig. 10-1).

The last step in localizing an aphasia-producing lesion requires that one consider two separate clinical parameters: fluency and auditory comprehension. Except for anomic aphasia, in which, by definition, language functions other than naming are spared, fluency and comprehension are often inversely related. Decreased fluency occurs with anterior (frontal) lesions of the language system, whereas poor comprehension follows posterior (temporal-parietal) damage. When both fluency and comprehension are impaired, the more global dysfunction suggests damage throughout the anterior-posterior extent of the language system. A fluent aphasia with good comprehension implies significant sparing of these two poles.

Fluency refers mainly to the ease of language production, but it implies more than this. Fluent speech is well articulated at a normal or even increased rate. Phrases are of normal length. Intonations and inflections are intact, and to a foreigner who did not know the language, a fluent aphasic might not even appear to have a speech disturbance. Fluent speech, however, may be devoid of words that convey meaning (such as nouns and verbs), or these "content" words may be used incorrectly (paraphasic errors).

In contrast, the initiation of nonfluent speech is impaired; it is effortfully and slowly produced, and phrases may be limited to one or two words. Speech may be dysarthric, and the normal melody of speech is lost. Because content words are often spared in preference to words whose function is primarily grammatical, such as prepositions and articles, nonfluent speech can still convey considerable information. Fluency is dependent upon the integrity of the anterior portion of the language system, and frontal lobe lesions within this system cause nonfluent aphasias.

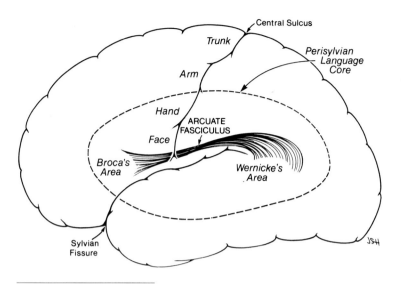

FIGURE 10-1.

Comprehension is not a unitary process, but the bedside evaluation of auditory comprehension usually focuses on the comprehension of content words. For example, a patient may be asked to answer simple questions ("Are you in bed?"), to point to various objects by name ("Show me the mirror") or functional description ("Show me where you might see your reflection"), or to follow serial commands ("Tear this piece of paper into two pieces. Put one piece in your pocket, and throw the other on the floor"). Comprehension may be disturbed by injury anywhere in the language system, but damage to temporal-parietal regions that include Wernicke's area impairs comprehension of content word meaning to a much greater extent than does frontal injury alone.

**W**hat is the anatomic diagnosis?

The patient is anomic and his repetition is impaired. We have already concluded that he has a left hemisphere cortical lesion within the perisylvian core of the language system. However, both comprehension and fluency are preserved, and Wernicke's and Broca's areas are, therefore, intact. This patient's lesion must lie between these two poles, disconnecting anterior and posterior language regions. A fluent, paraphasic aphasia with impaired repetition and normal comprehension is characteristic of conduction aphasia. Lesions producing conduction aphasia occur in either the temporal or parietal perisylvian region and extend subcortically to include the arcuate fasciculus (Fig. 10-1). Conduction aphasia may occur without accompanying neurologic signs, as with this patient. Depending on the extent of injury, there could also be visual field defects, sensory impairments, pyramidal tract signs, or a mild impairment in auditory comprehension. Table 10-1 summarizes findings in other types of aphasia.

**W**hat is the likely pathologic differential diagnosis of the patient's aphasia? In view of the patient's history and physical findings, refine the pathologic differential diagnosis into a neurologic differential diagnosis.

Table 10-1.
Acquired language disorders (aphasia)

| Aphasic Syndrome | Naming (language system) | Repetition (perisylvian core) | Fluency (anterior) | Comprehension (posterior) |
|---|---|---|---|---|
| Anomic | I | N | N | N |
| Broca's | I | I | I | N |
| Conduction | I | I | N | N |
| Wernicke's | I | I | N | I |
| Global | I | I | I | I |
| Transcortical motor | I | N | I | N |
| Transcortical sensory | I | N | N | I |
| Mixed transcortical | I | N | I | I |

I = impaired; N = normal or almost normal.

As discussed previously, the pathologic differential diagnosis for a discrete abnormality of a portion of the left cerebral cortex is that of focal lesions of the brain and its adjacent coverings. The abrupt onset of this patient's persistent conduction aphasia strongly implies a vascular cause (stroke) as the leading possibility in the neurologic differential diagnosis. Seizures and trauma also cause sudden neurologic symptoms, but with seizures the deficits are relatively transient and for trauma the inciting event is usually obvious.

Strokes are due to blood vessel rupture (hemorrhage) or occlusion (infarction) (Table 10-2). The absence of headache and other signs of increased intracranial pressure and of signs of meningeal irritation make intracranial hemorrhage unlikely. Therefore, the leading possibility in the differential diagnosis is an infarction.

The history of a recent heart attack suggests the cause for this patient's stroke. Shortly after a heart attack, blood clots may adhere to the damaged endocardial surface. Later, these clots may dislodge, traveling through the systemic circulation until they block smaller arteries elsewhere in the body. In the brain, these clots, or emboli, prevent blood flow, leading to the death of more distal neural tissue and causing symptoms appropriate to the distribution of the blocked vessel. Other cardiac conditions predisposing to blood clots and embolic stroke are arrhythmias (particularly atrial fibrillation) and valvular damage, such as occurs with rheumatic heart disease. In addition, certain congenital heart defects that allow venous blood to enter the arterial circulation (for example, ventricular septal defect) will permit clots from elsewhere in the body to reach the brain.

CT scan showed a lucent lesion involving the cortex and white matter of the inferior left parietal lobe. The neurologic diagnosis is embolic infarction.

Table 10-2.
Causes of stroke

*In the brain parenchyma*
- Arterial
  - Rupture
    - Hypertensive hemorrhage (rupture of small arteries into basal ganglia, thalamus, subcortical white matter, pons, or cerebellum)
    - Other (trauma, arteriovenous malformation, tumor, vasculitis)
  - Occlusion
    - Large arteries
      - Atherosclerosis (artery to artery embolization of atheromatous material or thrombus from site of atherosclerotic buildup)
      - Embolus from systemic circulation
        - Thrombus from heart (atrial fibrillation, valvular heart disease, mural thrombus after myocardial infarction)
        - Paradoxical embolus (congenital heart disease)
        - Other (tumor, foreign body, fat or air embolus with trauma)
      - Thrombosis (polycythemia vera, thrombocytosis, hyperviscosity, homocysteinuria, hemoglobinopathies and other coagulopathies, trauma, vasculitis, infection [meningitis, syphilis, mucormyscosis, malaria])
    - Small arteries
      - Lacunar strokes in hypertension (basal ganglia, thalamus, internal capsule and other subcortical white matter, pons, cerebellum)
      - Vasculitis
- Venous (e.g., superior sagittal sinus thrombosis associated with infection, tumor, coagulopathies, vasculitis, dehydration, childbirth, oral contraceptives)

*In the subarachnoid space (hemorrhage)*
- Aneurysm (most common: berry aneurysm)
- Arteriovenous malformation
- Other (trauma, vasculitis, septic embolism, venous thrombosis)

*In the subdural space (hemorrhage, usually caused by trauma)*

*In the extradural space (hemorrhage, usually caused by trauma)*

# Case 11

# Left-Sided Weakness and Perceptual Disturbances

## Case 11

A 47-year-old right-handed master carpenter, fired from his job because of "sloppy work," was hospitalized after a single generalized tonic clonic seizure. His wife reported that he had lost 10 pounds over the previous month and had been experiencing night sweats. For 2 weeks he had complained of head pain. To further inquiries about his illness, he replied that he had come to the hospital only to accompany his wife during her annual checkup.

He was a thin man with temperature of 38°C and pulse of 120 beats per minute. A diastolic murmur was heard along the left sternal border. When the examiner was sitting to the patient's left side, the patient was inattentive to the examiner's questions and looked to the right when responding, but he answered promptly whent he examiner moved to the patient's right side. Speech was flat (i.e., relatively monotonal) but well articulated and fluent, without word-finding difficulty or paraphasic errors. He was unable to put on his bathrobe; one sleeve was inside out, and, rather than invert it, he attempted to don the robe backward.

Visual fields were full to confrontation testing and acuity was normal, but he failed to detect finger movements in his left visual field when the examiner wiggled fingers in both fields simultaneously (i.e., visual extinction to double simultaneous stimulation). The left nasolabial fold was slightly flattened. He rarely moved his left limbs spontaneously. Mild left-sided weakness, hypertonia, hyperreflexia, and Babinski's sign were present. Sensation was normal to testing except that pinprick felt less sharp over his left side. With his eyes closed, he consistently failed to detect left-sided tactile stimuli when he was simultaneously touched on both the left and right sides (i.e., left-sided tactile extinction to double simultaneous stimulation). Perception of two-point discrimination was 5 mm on the ball of his right thumb (normal) but 15 mm on the left. With eyes closed, he identified numbers traced in his right hand but was often incorrect in his left hand.

In describing a picture from a magazine, he gave an accurate account of the right-hand portion of the scene but omitted details from the left. Simple line drawings were poorly executed. Individual components were not integrated into the overall design, and the left sides of his drawings remained incomplete, as when he attempted to copy a drawing of a daisy (Fig. 11-1A). When asked to draw the face of a clock, he placed all the numbers on the right side (Fig. 11-1B).

Damage to what systems caused the patient's left-sided weakness and sensory findings? What is their anatomy?

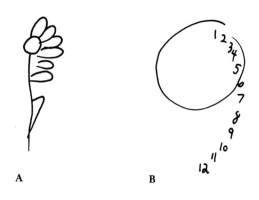

A    B

FIGURE 11-1.

## Case 11

The mild left-sided weakness, hypertonia, hyperreflexia, and Babinski's sign imply a lesion of the right corticospinal pathway. This pathway arises largely from the motor area of the right cerebral cortex; descends through the right internal capsule, cerebral peduncle, and basis pontis; crosses to the left side in the decussation of the medullary pyramids; and travels in the left lateral funiculus of the spinal cord to synapse on the anterior horn cell in the ventral gray region of the spinal cord (solid line, Fig. 11-2). As mild left-sided signs involve the face, as well as the arm and leg, the patient's corticospinal dysfunction must be rostral to the facial nucleus in the pons. However, more information is necessary to refine the anatomic diagnosis.

Elementary tactile sensation is almost normal. The patient's perception that pinprick seems less sharp over the left side of his face and limbs might represent a subtle disturbance in modalities mediated by the spinothalamic functional system. The spinothalamic tracts convey sensations of pain and light touch from the limbs through the contralateral spinal cord to the thalamus (Fig. 11-2, dashed line). Fibers of the trigeminal nerve, conveying facial sensation, course near the spinothalamic tract within the pons, medulla, and upper cervical spinal cord (dotted line, Fig. 11-2). The decreased pinprick sensation in the left upper and lower extremities and left side of the face implies a lesion after the second-order neurons have crossed to the right side. Spinothalamic system involvement, if present, must be above the level of the pons, since both the left face and body are involved.

However, there were more pronounced and qualitatively different sensory findings. This patient performed poorly on tasks such as two-point discrimination, graphesthesia (recognizing letters or numbers traced over the skin), and double simultaneous stimulation. The last impairment occurred with visual as well as tactile stimuli, implying that disturbances are not solely those of elementary sensory functional systems.

What anatomic diagnosis would account for these other sensory abnormalities?

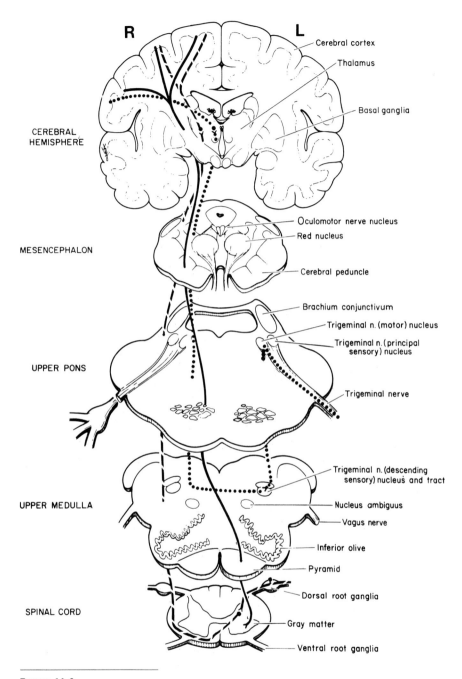

FIGURE 11-2.
Solid line: corticospinal tract; dotted line: spinothalamic fibers from face; dashed line: corticospinal fibers from body.

This type of sensory loss follows damage to parietal regions that integrate elementary sensory input and represents an impairment of discriminative, or cortical, sensation. These discriminative sensations include two-point discrimination, cutaneous stimulus localization (with the eyes closed, identifying the precise location of a tactile stimulus), graphesthesia, stereognosis (identifying objects by palpation alone), baroreception (discrimination of weight), and detection of simultaneously presented bilateral stimuli. Proprioceptive loss may also be marked after cortical damage. Cortical sensory disturbances are indicative of a cortical lesion and can occur even when elementary sensation is preserved, but usually some elevation in sensory threshold for touch and pinprick is present over the contralateral limbs. Cortical sensation, which depends on complex temporal and spatial integration, would then be more impaired than could readily be attributed to these relatively mild elementary deficits. In contrast, for sensory loss caused by lesions lower in the nervous system, the extent of the cortical sensory disturbance is predicated on the degree of more elementary deficits. Severe loss of any of the elementary sensations (touch, pain, temperature, and vibration) implies damage of the thalamus, brainstem, or below. Total absence of elementary sensations does not occur with lesions above the thalamus.

The parietal lobes not only contain the somatosensory cortex but also are involved in associations among several sensory modalities. Parietal lesions, particularly those of the inferior parietal lobe (supramarginal and angular gyri), therefore cause higher level perceptual deficits not limited to tactile modalities. Thus, this patient was impaired on tasks of double simultaneous stimulation for visual as well as tactile stimuli. Human perceptual and attentional deficits are especially severe after right-sided cerebral injury, suggesting that in people the right parietal lobe is relatively dominant for these functions. Similar but milder clinical findings are sometimes seen after lesions in other left and right hemisphere areas. Marked perceptual and attentional disturbances, which characterize extensive right parietal damage, are referred to as the neglect syndrome. Such persons may also fail to convey emotions by the tone of their voice or fail to understand emotional overtones in the speech of others.

This patient's perceptual difficulties are manifested by his drawings and by his inability to dress himself. Inattention, more pronounced for contralateral space, is reflected in both his drawing performance and in his response to people, objects, and other stimuli on his left. In addition, he consistently uses his right limbs preferentially, even though left-sided strength was but slightly reduced. Finally, he is unconcerned about these problems and explicitly denies the severity of his disability. In fact, he confabulates that his visit to the hospital is only to accompany his wife.

**What is the pathologic differential diagnosis? What are the most likely possibilities that constitute the neurologic differential diagnosis?**

The patient was hospitalized because of an acute symptom, a seizure, but his occupational history suggests that other symptoms and signs antedated the first manifestation of epilepsy. His seizure is, thus, likely a symptom of an underlying, insidiously progressive, irritative cortical lesion. Gradually, progressive neurologic symptoms are seen with expanding masses (e.g., tumors, abscesses), certain hereditary or degenerative disorders, "slow" viral infections, and toxins.

Focal damage to the cerebral hemispheres can derive from intrinsic or extrinsic elements. The slow development of focal damage is often caused by glial or metastatic neoplasms or by certain types of focal infections (granulomatous infections, abscesses). The patient's history of night sweats and weight loss and the findings of hyperthermia and of a heart murmur suggest infectious endocarditis. Endocarditis predisposes to intracranial infections. Thus, the neurologic differential diagnosis includes abscess and septic emboli. The history of headache is more consistent with abscess. A right parietal abscess was substantiated by CT scan and cerebral angiography and was verified during surgery. Endocarditis was confirmed by echocardiography and bacterial cultures of blood.

**Case 12**

**Right Visual Field Loss and Alexia**

## Case 12

One morning a 68-year-old well-educated right-handed businessman was astonished to discover that he was unable to read his newspaper. He denied other visual symptoms, understood what others said, and had no difficulty speaking. There were no disturbances of strength, sensation, coordination, or walking.

He was alert and oriented. There was a right homonymous hemianopsia (Fig. 12-1). Other cranial nerve functions were normal, as were strength, coordination, tendon reflexes, sensation, and gait. Speech was fluent, well articulated, and without paraphasic errors. Oral comprehension was normal. He was unable to name letters on the vision chart, but his responses indicated that his visual acuity was normal. For example, he described the letter A on the chart as a "sawhorse," Z as a "snake," and P as a "loop." To dictation, he wrote accurately, but shortly thereafter he was unable to read any of what he had written.

This patient presents two major findings. Vision is impaired in his right visual field in both eyes (Fig. 12-1), and he is unable to read (i.e., he is alexic). The former neurologic impairment is perhaps more straightforward. Damage to what region of the visual system produces a right homonymous hemianopsia?

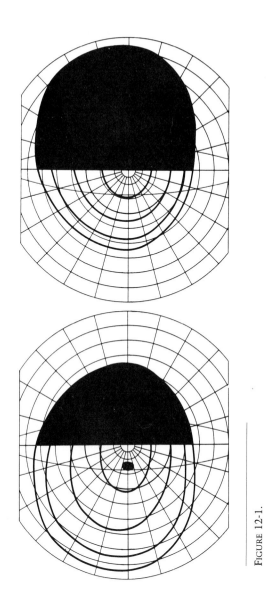

FIGURE 12-1.

As discussed previously, fibers from retinal ganglion cells located in the nasal (medial) portion of each retina cross the sagittal plane at the optic chiasm (Fig. 12-2). After the chiasm, the left optic tract thus contains fibers from the nasal (medial) half of the right retina and the temporal (lateral) half of the left retina. Visual information from the right visual field of each eye is thereby conveyed solely to the left cerebral hemisphere, and vice versa. Injury to visual fibers at any point distal to the chiasm causes homonymous field defects. A right homonymous hemianopsia might follow damage to the left optic tract, the left lateral geniculate nucleus of the thalamus where retinal ganglion cell axons terminate, the optic radiation (axons of lateral geniculate neurons, which course within the subcortical white matter of the left temporal and parietal lobes), or the primary visual cortex of the left occipital lobe (Fig. 12-2).

Language disturbances are caused by left hemisphere injury (see case 10). However, this patient's language impairments are quite circumscribed: Reading is impossible, but oral language (both speech and comprehension) is entirely normal, as is writing to dictation. The left hemisphere perisylvian language core is therefore intact. Patients with an isolated homonymous hemianopsia are usually able to read, so the loss of a visual field does not account for alexia if visual information from the intact hemifield can reach left hemisphere language areas. Involvement of what additional system is necessary to explain the patient's alexia?

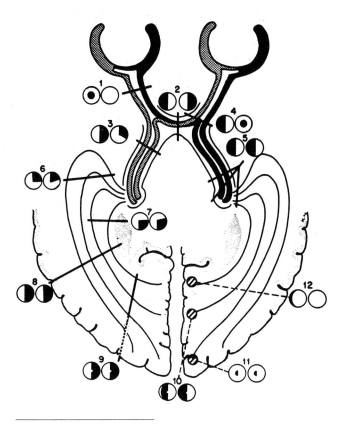

FIGURE 12-2.
Reproduced with permission from Harrington, D. O. *The Visual Fields* (5th ed.). St. Louis: Mosby, 1981.

Language functions depend on integrity of left hemisphere language areas. Significant damage to this region should impair all aspects of language: spoken language, speech comprehension, reading, and writing. This patient, however, has "pure" alexia (also referred to as alexia without agraphia): In the absence of other language abnormalities, he fails to understand what he reads. We must conclude that left hemisphere language areas are intact but that visual information is disconnected from posterior language areas responsible for language comprehension.

For any right homonymous hemianopsia, there is no direct visual input into the language dominant left hemisphere. Rather, reading requires that visual information first be transmitted to the left hemisphere from the visual association cortex of the right hemisphere. Most interhemispheric transfer involves the corpus callosum, the massive white matter bundle that facilitates interhemispheric functional integration by linking certain cortical association areas of the two cerebral hemispheres. Empirically, it is known that visual input processed occipitally crosses to the contralateral hemisphere via the posterior portion of the corpus callosum, a region known as the splenium. The anatomic lesion producing this patient's pure alexia is therefore one that both causes his right homonymous hemianopsia and also interrupts crossing callosal fibers conveying contralateral visual input to posterior left hemisphere language areas.

The lesion that usually causes pure alexia is shown in the shaded area of Figure 12-3. Damage to the calcarine cortex of the left occipital lobe, of course, accounts for the right homonymous hemianopsia. The area of injury also included crossing fibers in the splenium of the corpus callosum, thereby precluding right hemisphere visual input from reaching posterior left hemisphere language areas.

The pathologic differential diagnosis is that described earlier for a focal cerebral hemispheric lesion. Symptom onset was abrupt, suggesting a vascular cause as opposed to a slowly expanding mass lesion, such as a tumor. The anatomic location of the lesion corresponds to the area of brain supplied by the left posterior cerebral artery. Thus, the neurologic diagnosis is infarction in the distribution of the left posterior cerebral artery.

This patient's case description is adapted from one originally reported almost a century ago by the French neurologist Jules Dejerine. From previous studies Dejerine already knew that the left angular gyrus in the inferior parietal lobe was a language area crucial for the comprehension of visual language. Direct damage to the left angular gyrus can cause the clinical syndrome of alexia with agraphia. Both reading and writing are markedly impaired, whereas the oral language disturbance, often limited to anomia, is less prominent.

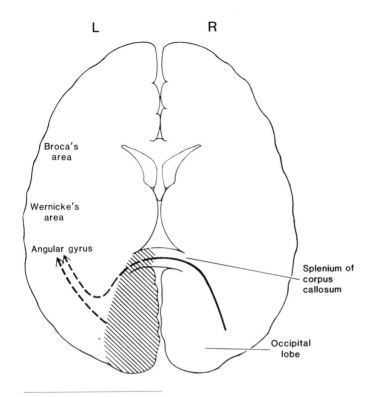

FIGURE 12-3.

Though uncommon, pure alexia is the prototype of a group of disorders referred to as hemisphere disconnection syndromes. Symptoms occur because one region of the cerebral cortex is isolated, or disconnected, from another. For the present case of pure alexia, left occipital and splenium damage precluded visual input from reaching the left hemisphere language areas. For other patients, a strategically located lesion within the white matter of the left parietal lobe might undercut the angular gyrus to produce symptoms of pure alexia with or without an accompanying visual field defect.

A partial list of hemispheric disconnection syndromes is given in Table 12-1. For some, a simple white matter disconnection hypothesis is undoubtedly an oversimplification of symptom pathogenesis, but the concept of intrahemispheric and interhemispheric disconnection is heuristically valuable for the clinician.

Reading is occasionally impaired by right hemisphere damage. Here, the disturbance is not due to a language disorder but is caused by severe impairments in visuospatial perception. Omissions and errors in reading are confined to the initial (left-sided) portion of sentences or individual words even if there is no associated hemianopsia. For example, *baseball* may be read as "ball" and *clover* as "lover" or "over." Words written vertically are correctly read, and speech (oral language) is normal. Because of other symptoms and signs of right hemisphere damage, these patients are rarely mistaken as having alexia from left hemisphere injury.

When the medical and social histories are not assiduously obtained, the inexperienced clinician might also mistake illiteracy for alexia. Patients unable to read because of educational impoverishment, mental retardation, or developmental learning disorders should not be categorized as alexic. Table 12-2 gives a simple classification of reading disorders. (Other modern classification schemes are based on linguistic analyses as to the type of reading error.)

Table 12-1.
Hemisphere disconnection syndromes

| Syndrome | Functional Areas Disconnected | Lesion Location |
| --- | --- | --- |
| Pure alexia | Angular gyrus/visual cortex | Left occipital lobe, splenium of corpus callosum |
| Conduction aphasia | Broca's area/Wernicke's area | Arcuate fasciculus |
| Mixed transcortical aphasia | Left hemisphere auditory cortex and perisylvian language core/rest of cortex | Arterial borderzone in frontal, parietal, temporal lobes |
| Pure word deafness | Wernicke's area/auditory cortex | Left subtemporal lesion undercutting Wernicke's area  Lesions of both temporal lobes |
| Sympathetic apraxia | Right premotor and motor cortex/Wernicke's area | Broca's area, anterior corpus callosum |

Table 12-2.
Reading disorders

*Acquired reading disorders (alexia)*
  Associated with left hemisphere damage
    Pure alexia (alexia without agraphia)
    Alexia with agraphia
    Aphasic alexia
  Associated with right hemisphere damage and the neglect syndrome
*Developmental reading disorders (dyslexia)*
*Illiteracy*

# Case 13

# Speech Difficulty, Right-Sided Weakness, and Clumsiness of the Left Hand

## Case 13

A 60-year-old right-handed man returned for follow-up evaluation. A month before, when he tried to get out of bed, he was unable to walk because of weakness of the right leg. He could not move his right arm, and, according to his wife, the right corner of his mouth drooped. The patient was unable to speak, but his wife said he understood much of what she told him as she drove him to the hospital. He denied visual and sensory disturbances. Over the next several weeks speech and right-sided weakness slowly improved.

During the preceding year there had been two episodes of transient visual loss of the left eye, "like a shade was being pulled down," each lasting 20 minutes and gradually resolving over 5 minutes.

On examination the right nasolabial fold was flattened and the right palpebral fissure was widened, but each side of the forehead wrinkled normally. Other cranial nerve functions were intact, as was tactile sensation. The right upper extremity was flexed and plegic. In the right lower extremity extensor tone was increased, and there was mild weakness. On the left side strength was normal, as were rapid alternating movements and coordination on the finger-to-nose and heel-knee-shin tasks. On the right, tendon reflexes were abnormally brisk and Babinski's sign was present. As he walked, there was circumduction of the extended right leg.

Spontaneous speech was poorly articulated. Consonants were slurred, and speech was slowly produced with great effort. The underlying melody or cadence was lost, and speech was thus monotonal. His speech was limited to single words and short phrases, but he nevertheless conveyed considerable information. For example, when asked to describe his illness, he replied, "One month, stroke. Wife...drove...car...hospital. Better now." There were few paraphasic errors. Although still somewhat slurred, speech was more easily produced and melody was better as he counted from 1 to 10. His ability to understand others' speech was satisfactory for routine conversation. He had moderate difficulty providing names for common objects shown to him, and he could not accurately repeat phrases or sentences.

Despite understanding the task, he was unable to carry out certain requested activities with his left hand. For example, when asked to pretend to brush his teeth, he rubbed his left hand over his face and mouth. However, when given his toothbrush, he performed the task correctly, thus demonstrating that strength and coordination were not limiting his performance on his previous attempt. He had similar difficulty executing commands that involved facial, oral, and respiratory musculature. When asked to cough, he said "uh . . . uh . . . cough," cleared his throat, and stated, "Can't." He was later observed to cough spontaneously.

First, determine how this man's speech is affected. Is the speech disorder one of dysarthria, aphasia, or both?

Articulation is poor and thus, by definition, the patient is dysarthric. Dysarthria follows damage to a variety of neural and nonneural structures (Table 13-1). Lesions of the cerebral hemispheres, corticobulbar fibers, deep nuclear structures, brainstem, cerebellum, or facial, glossopharyngeal, vagus, or hypoglossal nerves impair articulation. Dysarthria also has causes as mundane as ill-fitting dentures or can be produced by injury to nonneural structures that are mechanically important in speech production, such as the tongue, palate, larynx, and muscles of respiration. Nasal obstruction imparts a nasal quality to speech.

Occasionally, other factors will affect speech. Lacking auditory feedback, deaf persons are often dysarthric. Stuttering sometimes follows central nervous system lesions but more typically begins in childhood in the absence of known structural abnormality.

The experienced clinician can distinguish several specific patterns of neurogenic dysarthria. Most are accompanied by other deficits of functional motor (or occasionally, sensory) systems.

Scanning dysarthria of cerebellar disease is characterized by uncoordinated breath control causing irregular, sometimes explosive, fluctuations in speech volume and rate. The slow, slurred speech of spastic dysarthria follows lesions of corticobulbar portions of the pyramidal motor system and is accompanied by brisk gag and facial reflexes and by slow tongue movements. For the parkinsonian patient with basal ganglia disease, rigidity and gait festination are paralleled by articulatory stiffness and "speech festination"—soft, monotonous mumbling, which increases in tempo and decreases in volume toward the end of a long sentence. The patient with parkinsonism exhibits a tendency to repeat individual syllables (palilalia)—which may reflect general difficulty in initiating new motor sequences—and, like the limbs, the voice is often tremulous. Dysarthria also accompanies hyperkinetic extrapyramidal disorders, such as the chorea of Huntington's disease.

Weakness of the bulbar musculature imparts a "denasal" quality to speech as excessive air escapes through the nose. Sounds requiring movement of the palate (K), tongue (L), or lips (M) are poorly articulated. When bulbar weakness is caused by disorders of the neuromuscular junction (for example, myasthenia gravis), this "flaccid" dysarthria will rapidly worsen as the patient fatigues.

Occasionally, two dysarthric patterns may occur in the same patient. For example, a person with amyotrophic lateral sclerosis, a disease affecting both lower and upper motoneurons, may have both denasal speech and signs of spastic dysarthria. The victim of multiple sclerosis, with axonal demyelination in several central nervous system sites, may have components of both spastic and cerebellar dysarthria.

From a written protocol, it is difficult to be certain as to the kind of dysarthria, but this patient's slow, slurred speech suggests spastic dysarthria caused by dysfunction of the corticobulbar system. This impression is reinforced by findings of corticospinal dysfunction: right-sided weakness, spasticity, hyperreflexia, and Babinski's sign. Together, these signs point to damage of the left corticospinal system.

Where within the corticospinal system is the lesion responsible for his motor disturbance?

Table 13-1.
Dysarthria—functional classification

| Type | Cause |
| --- | --- |
| Neurogenic dysarthria | |
|   Spastic dysarthria | Corticobulbar lesions |
|   Extrapyramidal dysarthria | Basal ganglia lesions |
|   Scanning dysarthria | Lesions of the cerebellum or its connections |
|   Flaccid dysarthria | Lower motor neuron, neuromuscular junction, or peripheral nerve lesions |
|   Sensory dysarthria | Usually peripheral nerve lesions |
|   Mixed dysarthria | Combination of above lesions |
| Nonneurogenic dysarthria | Injury to tongue, palate, larnynx, muscles of respiration, etc. |

Right-sided weakness includes the face, arm, and leg. Right facial weakness is that of an upper motoneuron lesion: Muscles of the forehead are relatively spared, whereas weakness of muscles about the eye and mouth leads to widening of the right palpebral fissure and drooping of the right nasolabial fold. The left corticospinal lesion, affecting fibers to the contralateral face, arm, and leg, must therefore lie above the level of the pons (see case 2).

Within the brainstem and internal capsule, corticospinal fibers partially intermingle and are tightly packed into a small area. Corticospinal fibers originate from a much larger area in the cerebral cortex (Fig. 13-1). Lesions in the internal capsule ordinarily affect the contralateral face, arm, and leg to a similar degree. With small cortical lesions, the face and arm may be involved more than the leg (middle cerebral artery territory), or the leg may be more involved than the arm and face (anterior cerebral artery territory). For this patient, right leg paresis is milder than the complete paralysis of the right upper extremity—suggesting cortical involvement.

In addition to trouble with articulation, the patient also has difficulty with language production. What anatomic diagnosis within the functional language system accounts for his aphasia? Consider first whether or not the perisylvian language core is affected.

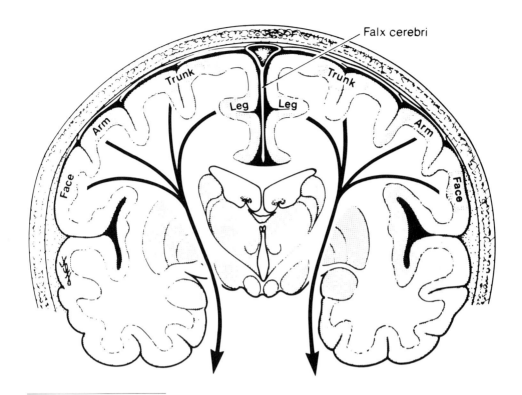

Figure 13-1.

## Case 13

As noted earlier, for right-handers aphasia is almost always due to injury to the left cerebral hemisphere. Word-finding difficulty (anomia), occurring in this patient's spontaneous speech and on a task of visual confrontation naming, confirms that a language disturbance is present but is of little localizing value within the left hemisphere language system. His problem in repeating verbatim the examiner's phrases, however, tells us that the anatomic disturbance involves the perisylvian language core (Fig. 13-2).

The next step in localization is to decide whether the perisylvian lesion is predominantly anterior or posterior to the central sulcus. When one considers both speech fluency and comprehension—clinical parameters that are important for this determination—what is the anatomic diagnosis for his aphasia?

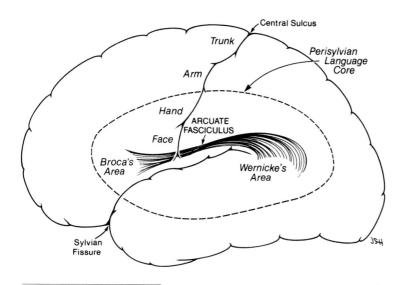

FIGURE 13-2.

His speech is produced effortfully, and the underlying melody is lost. Phrase length and speech rate are reduced. Because the patient's speech includes many meaningful content words (nouns, verbs, adjectives), he manages to convey a great deal of information. There are few paraphasic errors.

These features typify nonfluent speech (see case 10) and indicate a lesion that includes the anterior speech areas. Since comprehension is relatively preserved, posterior language regions must be largely spared. Nonfluent speech with impaired repetition and good comprehension is characteristic of Broca's aphasia. The usual anatomic diagnosis is a left hemisphere lesion that includes Broca's area (shaded area, Fig. 13-3). Broca's area is contiguous to the anterior border of the lower left precentral gyrus, the origin of many of the corticobulbar and corticospinal fibers that constitute the pyramidal motor system. Thus, it is not surprising that Broca's aphasics also have a right hemiplegia.

There remains another clinical sign to be explained. With his left hand and arm, the patient is apraxic to command. Apraxia refers to the inability to execute simple commands even though strength, sensation, and coordination are adequate for the task and even though the patient understands the request and is motivated to accomplish it. Thus, when handed a toothbrush, the patient promptly demonstrated how to brush his teeth, using his nonparalyzed left upper extremity. Without the toothbrush, however, his left arm movements were again only a crude approximation of the target task.

Before any verbal command can be executed, verbal information must first be processed in the auditory cortex and in Wernicke's area. Damage to Wernicke's area would impair comprehension, and such patients should not be considered apraxic if they fail to understand the examiner's request. Similarly, injury to muscle, peripheral nerve axons, spinal cord or brainstem motor nuclei, or the upper motoneuron may cause paralysis, precluding execution of the command. However, hemisphere lesions that disconnect Wernicke's area from prefrontal and motor cortex sometimes will prevent the execution of an understood command by an otherwise functionally normal limb.

On the basis of these considerations, what anatomic lesion accounts for this patient's left upper extremity apraxia to command? Is there right hemisphere damage, or is the previous anatomic diagnosis sufficient to explain all the symptoms and signs?

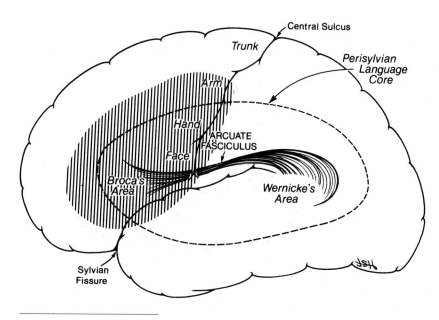

FIGURE 13-3.

Figure 13-4 schematically shows hypothetical pathways mediating a motor response to a verbal command. The verbal command is first processed in the primary auditory cortex of the temporal lobes and then in Wernicke's area in the adjacent left temporal lobe. Pathways (probably the arcuate fasciculus) link Wernicke's area with Broca's area and the left premotor cortex. For right arm movements, connection is then made with the ipsilateral motor cortex.

For commands executed by the left upper extremity, information regarding the task must reach the right hemisphere via the corpus callosum (Fig. 13-4). From these simple considerations, one can predict that subcortical injury that disconnects Wernicke's area from the frontal lobe will cause bilateral limb apraxia. As expected, many patients with conduction aphasia, who may have lesions within this area, are apraxic.

This patient has a right hemiparesis and Broca's aphasia. The expected anatomic location of his lesion (see Fig. 13-3) includes Broca's area and adjacent regions of the motor and premotor cortex. Such a lesion, affecting cells of origin for frontal transcallosal fibers as well as the fibers to the right upper extremity, will cause left upper extremity apraxia to command ("sympathetic" apraxia) and right upper extremity paralysis.

A similar explanation accounts for the oral-facial apraxia of many Broca's aphasics. (More precisely, the "oral-facial" apraxia involves the face, mouth, larynx, and muscles of respiration.) Such patients may be unable to cough on command or to execute commands such as "Show me how you would smell a rose." However, these patients will cough spontaneously and will be able to sniff when actually handed a rose.

The apraxias are assumed to result from interruptions between motor cortex and left hemisphere language areas. As such, apraxias are an example of the cortical disconnection syndromes discussed in case 12. However, this formulation does not explain all varieties of apraxia. For right-handers, the left hemisphere is specialized not only for language functions but also for skilled motor movements, such as the fine movements of which the fingers are capable. Unilateral motor specialization may account for some forms of apraxia not explicable in terms of a disconnection hypothesis.

This patient has a past history of transient monocular loss of vision (amaurosis fugax) on the left side. What does the history of amaurosis fugax suggest as to pathologic and neurologic differential diagnoses for this patient's right hemiparesis, Broca's aphasia, dysarthria, and apraxia?

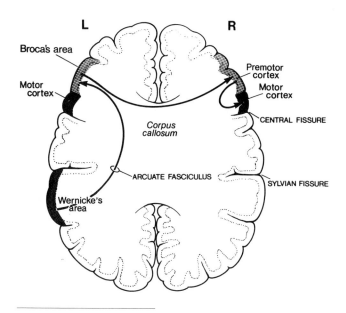

FIGURE 13-4.

The pathologic differential diagnosis for focal cortical lesions has been discussed in previous cases. In narrowing the diagnostic possibilities for this patient, the past history of amaurosis fugax of the left eye suggests that he is predisposed to emboli originating from atherosclerosis of the left carotid artery. Amaurosis fugax is usually caused by a fragment of atherosclerotic plaque or small platelet-thrombin embolus, which temporarily blocks the central retinal artery, a branch of the ophthalmic artery. As the embolus disintegrates, blood flow is restored and vision returns. The ophthalmic artery is a branch of the internal carotid artery (Fig. 13-5). Emboli causing amaurosis fugax often arise from more proximal atherosclerotic changes, usually where the common carotid artery bifurcates into its internal and external branches. Both the left retina and the already established anatomic diagnosis for the patient's other symptoms are included in the vascular territory of the left internal carotid artery. Note, however, that his infarct does not involve the entire left carotid distribution; rather, only anterior branches of the left middle cerebral artery are occluded. Infarction in this distribution is a frequent cause of Broca's aphasia. Like other lesions causing persistent Broca's aphasia, the region is considerably larger than the discrete posterior portion of the left inferior frontal gyrus traditionally designated as Broca's area itself.

Similarly, persistent Wernicke's aphasia often follows a large infarct of the posterior left hemisphere and involves more posterior branches of the left middle cerebral artery. More extensive infarction from occlusion of the middle cerebral artery at its origin or of the entire left internal carotid usually causes global aphasia. Prolonged hypotension will selectively decrease perfusion of the most distal branches of the anterior, middle, and posterior cerebral arteries (watershed zone; see Fig. 13-5). The resulting border-zone infarction can cause a transcortical or isolation aphasia. (See Table 10-1.)

The most likely item in the neurologic differential diagnosis is infarction in the distribution of the anterior branches of the left middle cerebral artery, caused by emboli arising proximal to the ophthalmic artery, probably from an ulcerating atherosclerotic plaque at the bifurcation of the left common carotid.

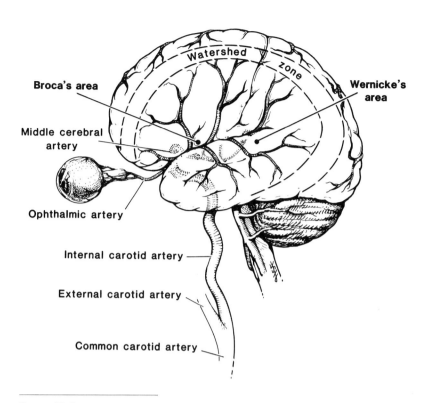

FIGURE 13-5.

# Case 14

# Gait and Truncal Ataxia and Headache

# Case 14

A 10-year-old boy was brought to the office because of increasing clumsiness. His mother noted that he walked as though he were drunk and that he occasionally fell. He would fall in any direction. His hands were not clumsy. The child's only other complaint was intermittent occipital head pain, which worsened when he coughed or bent over. These symptoms, first noticed 3 months earlier, had worsened progressively.

The child was alert, oriented, and cooperative. Speech was fluent and well articulated. Cranial nerve functions were normal. Sensation was intact to pinprick, light touch, proprioception, and vibration. Strength, muscle tone, and tendon reflexes were normal. The boy was able to move his index finger from his nose and to the examiner's finger (finger-nose-finger test) (Fig. 14-1A) without dysmetria (an error in judging distance of a movement), ataxia (incoordination), or tremor. There was no decomposition of movement (the breaking down of complex movements into a series of simpler movements). Rapid alternating movements of his upper extremities were normal (i.e., there was no dysdiadochokinesia). However, with both legs he had difficulty maintaining his heel on his shin when asked to place his heel on the opposite knee and run the heel smoothly down his shin (heel-knee-shin test) (Fig. 14-1B).

While sitting on the examining table, the boy tended to sway in all directions. He walked with a wide-based gait and staggered in all directions. He was unable to stand on either foot alone. When standing with his eyes open and feet together, he was able to maintain his balance for only a few seconds before swaying.

Involvement of what functional anatomic system explains the patient's gait disturbance?

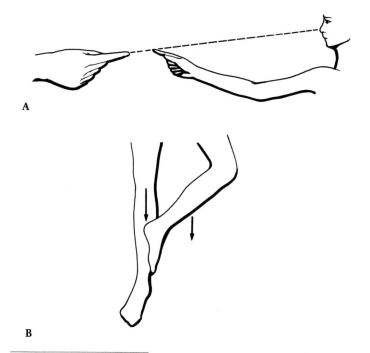

FIGURE 14-1.

The patient's dysfunction is limited to balance and lower extremity coordination. Both weakness and sensory loss can cause difficulty with balance and lower extremity use. However, his strength and sensation were normal. Spinal cord lesions of the dorsal columns that impair balance are associated with Romberg's sign, which is defined as increased sway when the patient stands with the feet together and eyes closed compared to when the eyes are open. In this case the instability was the same, eyes open or closed. The Romberg sign was, therefore, absent.

A cerebellar lesion would explain this patient's gait ataxia, truncal ataxia, and ataxia on the heel-knee-shin test. Yet, if this were the case, why were there no signs and symptions of cerebellar dysfunction in the patient's upper extremities or speech? Is there localization of function in the cerebellum such that a restricted lesion might cause this patient's symptoms and signs?

Functionally, the cerebellum is divided into three longitudinal zones: (1) the midline or vermal region (corresponding to the vermis in the midline of the cerebellum); (2) the intermediate or paravermal region; and (3) the lateral region (the cerebellar hemispheres, Fig. 14-2). These three zones are characterized by distinct projections to the deep cerebellar nuclei and in their projections to the rest of the nervous system. The midline zone has connections primarily with the spinal cord and vestibular system; the lateral zone with the cerebral cortex; and the intermediate zone with both spinal cord and cerebral cortex.

The basal portion of the cerebellum, the flocculonodular lobe, is an extension of the vestibular complex and is functionally separate from the remaining cerebellum. It has reciprocal connections with vestibular and reticular nuclei of the brainstem.

Lateral zone injury causes ataxia, tremor of the ipsilateral extremities, and cerebellar dysarthria. Lesions of the midline zone cause gait, but not upper limb, ataxia. Lesions of the intermediate zone may produce both gait, truncal, and limb ataxia. Lesions of the flocculonodular lobe cause truncal and gait ataxia.

In this case, speech and upper extremity coordination are normal. The lesion must therefore be confined to the midline zone of the cerebellum. What does this localization imply as to the pathologic and neurologic differential diagnosis?

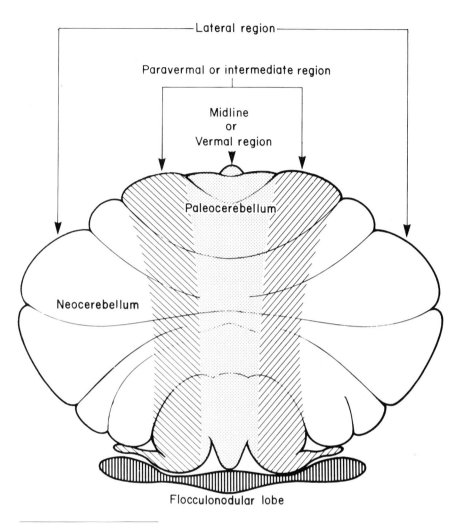

Figure 14-2.

Possibilities for the pathologic differential diagnosis include infarcts, tumors, abscesses, degenerative disorders, demyelination, and infections. Analysis of the history allows refinement of the pathologic differential diagnosis into a list of likely pathologic possibilities, i.e., the neurologic differential diagnosis. The patient had had headaches for 3 months; such an onset of headaches might suggest increased intracranial pressure from an expanding mass lesion. Coughing and bending increase intrathoracic and intraabdominal pressure, which is transmitted by the venous system to the cranial cavity. For this patient, worsening of the headaches with coughing or bending is further evidence of increased intracranial pressure.

The volume of the intracranial cavity is determined by the rigid skull. The contents of the skull can be divided into three components: (1) blood, (2) cerebrospinal fluid (CSF), and (3) brain (Fig. 14-3). An increase in any one of these increases intracranial pressure. For example, hemorrhage into the brain increases the blood component, thereby increasing intracranial pressure. Blockage of CSF flow and absorption increase the CSF component. Tumors, abscesses, and edema increase the brain component. The presence of increased intracranial pressure in this case favors certain pathologic possibilities. The gradual onset of the patient's headache suggests a slowly expanding lesion, such as tumor or abscess. Lesions that acutely increase intracranial pressure, such as a cerebellar hematoma or edema from an infarct, are therefore so improbable as to be virtually excluded from the neurologic differential diagnosis.

At this point, adjunctive laboratory tests are used for further determination of the neurologic differential diagnosis. CT scan of the head showed a mass in the midline of the cerebellum. In children such midline masses are apt to be tumors, particularly medulloblastomas. These tumors arise from primitive cells found in this region during prenatal and infant development. A diagnosis of a medulloblastoma was confirmed at surgery.

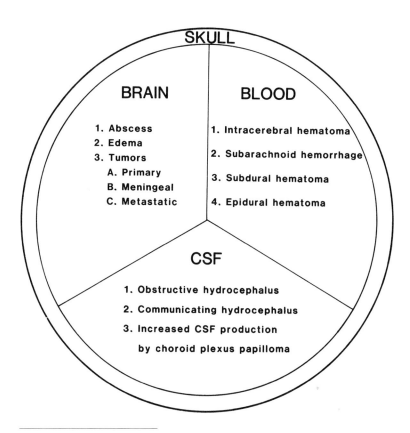

FIGURE 14-3.

**Case 15**

# Ataxia and Weakness of the Left Arm

## Case 15

A 53-year-old man came to the emergency room because of weakness and clumsiness of the left hand and arm, which had begun suddenly a few hours earlier. While walking, he noticed that he slightly dragged his left leg and stumbled, falling to the left side. His left hand became tremulous and unstable when he attempted to reach for a cup. He denied headache or changes in vision, sensation, or balance. He had a history of high blood pressure.

The patient's blood pressure was 190/110 mm Hg. His speech was fluent and well articulated. Cranial nerve functions were normal. Sensory examination revealed normal response to pinprick, light touch, vibration, proprioception, and double simultaneous stimulation. Tone was normal, but on the left side there was slight weakness of the hand grip, finger abductors and adductors, and hip flexors. Also on the left, ataxia and tremor were found on finger-nose-finger and heel-knee-shin testing, greater than what would be expected from the weakness alone. The tendon reflexes were hyperreflexic, and Babinski's sign was present on the left side.

Involvement of what functional system is causing the left-sided weakness? What is its anatomy? Next, determine what systems were involved in producing the ataxia and tremor. How are they related to the left-sided weakness? Figure 15-1 represents several sections through the CNS including the cerebellar cortex and deep cerebellar nuclei. The reader may wish to sketch the anatomy of the systems involved.

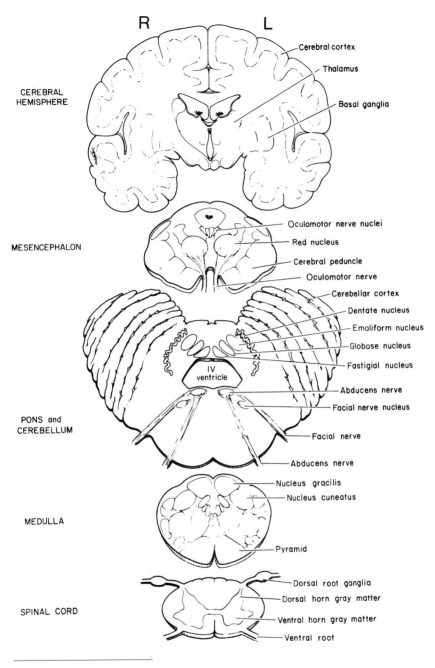

FIGURE 15-1.

## Case 15

As in the previous cases, weakness, hyperreflexia and Babinski's sign on the left side imply a lesion of the corticospinal pathway (solid line, Fig. 15-2). More data are needed for further localization of the lesion. More information can be obtained from an analysis of the left-sided ataxia and tremor.

Some patients with lesions of the corticospinal pathway (i.e., upper motoneuron syndrome) have ataxia and tremor due simply to weakness. However, in the case presented, the ataxia and tremor are disproportionate to what might be expected from the patient's slight weakness. Ataxia and tremor may also be associated with position sense loss, but none was found on examination of this patient.

The limb ataxia and tremor may be due to a lesion of the left lateral zone of the cerebellum (shaded area, Fig. 15-2). (Recall from case 14 that cerebellar lesions cause ipsilateral symptoms.) However, to explain the left-sided upper motoneuron findings, a single lesion would have to extend from the left cerebellum to the right basis pontis. Such a large lesion should affect other brainstem systems. However, in this case there are no other symptoms and signs of brainstem involvement.

How did the cerebellar symptoms and signs arise?

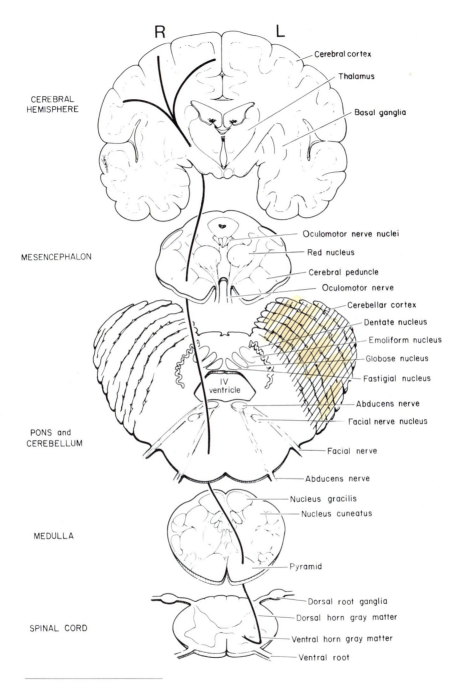

FIGURE 15-2.
Solid line: corticospinal tract.

Like lesions of the cerebellum itself, a lesion of the efferent or afferent connections to the lateral zone of the cerebellum may cause signs similar to lesions of the cerebellum itself. The cerebellar cortex and the dentate nucleus of the lateral zone of the cerebellum receive projections from wide areas of the contralateral cerebral cortex. These fibers, which run through the internal capsule and cerebral peduncle, synapse on the pontine nuclei (dashed line, Fig. 15-3). Fibers arise from the pontine nuclei, cross the basis pontis, and ascend to the cerebellum through the middle cerebellar peduncle, or brachium pontis. The cerebellum also receives projections from the inferior olivary complex (not shown).

The output of the lateral zone originates in the dentate nucleus (dotted line, Fig. 15-3). Fibers travel from the dentate nucleus via the brachium conjunctivum, which decussates just caudal to the red nucleus and ascends to synapse in the ventroanterior and ventrolateral thalamus. From the ventroanterior and ventrolateral thalamus fibers ascend to motor areas of the cerebral cortex (Fig. 15-3). The lesion in this case must involve either the descending corticopontocerebellar fibers or the brachium conjunctivum, on the same side of the midbrain as the involved corticospinal fibers. For the latter, the lesion would have to be in the midbrain rostral to the decussation of the brachium conjunctivum, since the cerebellar signs are on the same side as the corticospinal signs. The lesion would also have to be caudal to the level of the thalamus where the corticospinal fibers and brachium conjunctivum are separate. Such a single lesion would be expected to include other interposed structures such as the oculomotor nerve. The lesion could be in the cerebral cortex, corona radiata, internal capsule, or basis pontis affecting the corticospinal fibers and corticopontocerebellar fibers. However, lesions of the cerebral cortex or corona radiata often cause other findings, such as sensory loss.

The two remaining possibilities are lesions of the internal capsule or of the basis pontis (ventral pons). These two possibilities may be difficult to distinguish. The fact that both sides of the face move fully suggests that the lesion is caudal to where the corticobulbar fibers to the face nuclei have separated from the corticospinal fibers. This formulation supports the basis pontis as the anatomic diagnosis.

Consider the anatomic diagnosis and the patient's history. What is the pathologic differential diagnosis? Which are the more likely diagnostic possibilities (i.e., the neurologic differential diagnosis)?

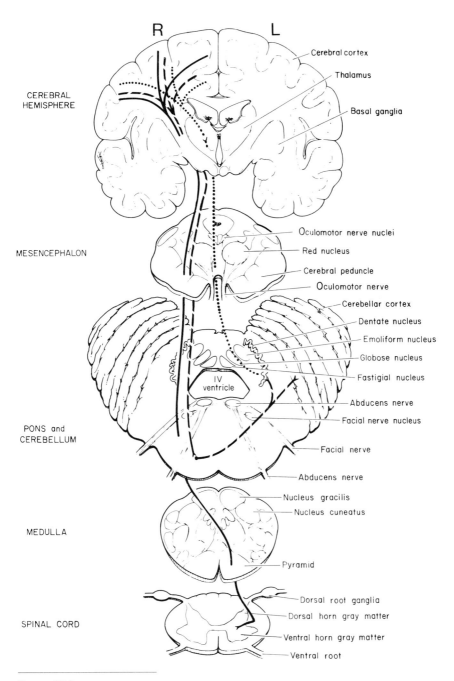

FIGURE 15-3.
Solid line: corticospinal tract; dashed line: fronto-ponto-cerebellar tract; dotted line: dentato-thalamo-cortical tract.

As discussed earlier, the sudden onset of symptoms is often due to a stroke. In the absence of evidence by history or examination of a space-occupying lesion, cerebral vascular disease is most likely. Different arteries supply different regions of the brain as shown in Fig 15-4 (1: anterior cerebral; 2: middle cerebral; 3: posterior cerebral; 4: superior cerebellar; 5,8,11: short circumferential branches; 7,10: long circumferential branches; 6,9: posterior inferior cerebellar; 12: posterior spinal; 13: anterior spinal. If the disorder in this case is occlusion of a large artery to the brain, then the anatomic localization should be consistent with that artery's territory. It can be seen from Fig 15-4 that the anatomic lesion does not conform to the vascular territory of a major arterial system.

Occlusion of a major branch of the basilar artery would probably cause a large lesion involving more functional systems than in this patient. Infarction from occlusion of small end arteries may cause the symptoms and signs he exhibited. These small infarcts are called lacunar infarcts. A small hemorrhage is also possible, but this possibility was excluded by the absence of fresh blood on CT scan.

Lacunae are infarcts from occlusion of the small end arteries. They measure about 0.5 to 1.5 cm in diameter and usually occur in hypertensive patients in specific regions of the brain. Lacunar infarcts are associated with characteristic clinical syndromes but of course are not the only cause of these syndromes. Table 15-1 lists the more common sites of lacunar infarcts and the associated clinical signs.

Table 15.1.
Common sites of lacunar infarcts and associated syndromes

| Site | Clinical Syndromes |
| --- | --- |
| Thalamus | Sensory loss of contralateral face, trunk, and extremities |
| Internal capsule | Weakness of contralateral face, trunk, and extremities, with or without ataxia; or contralateral sensory loss |
| Ventral pons | Weakness of contralateral extremities with or without ataxia; clumsy hand-dysarthria syndrome |
| Corona radiata | Weakness of contralateral face, trunk, and extremities, with or without ataxia; or contralateral sensory loss |
| Diffuse multiple sites | "Multi-infarct" dementia; pseudobulbar palsy |

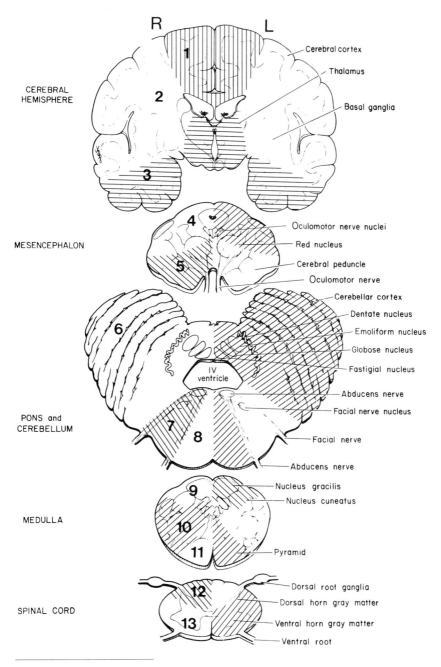

FIGURE 15-4.

**Case 16**

**Unconsciousness, Left-Sided Weakness, and Dysconjugate Gaze**

## Case 16

A 74-year-old man with a history of hypertension was brought to the emergency room by his daughter, who had found him unconscious on his bedroom floor. When she visited him the day before, he had appeared well.

In the emergency room the patient's vital signs were normal. He was lying quietly on the stretcher with his eyes closed. He occasionally moved his right extremities. The left lower extremity was externally rotated at the hip. With expiration the right cheek appeared to puff out more than the left, and his right forehead appeared less furrowed. The patient did not respond to his name being called or to being shaken. When pricked with a pin on either side of the body, he grimaced and attempted to fend off the stimulus with his right upper extremity. In grimacing, only the left corner of the mouth elevated. When the eyelids were held open, the right eye deviated to the left (Fig. 16-1), while the left eye stared straight ahead. When the head was quickly rotated to the left (oculocephalic or doll's-head maneuver), the right eye moved to the midline and stopped, and the left eye moved fully to the right. Both eyes moved conjugately to the left when the head was quickly turned to the right. When the head was rotated up and down, both eyes appropriately moved in the opposite direction (i.e., vertical eye movements were intact). There was eyelid closure on the left but not on the right side when either the right or left cornea was touched. The gag reflex was present on both sides. On the left side, tone was increased, tendon reflexes were brisk, and Babinski's sign was present.

The patient has a decreased level of consciousness. What are the structures necessary for consciousness? What does this imply in terms of the anatomic diagnosis?

**R**                **L**

Head straight

Head turned left

Head turned right

FIGURE 16-1.

When patients are unable to give a history or cooperate with the examination, neurologic diagnosis may seem difficult. However, much pertinent information can be obtained by careful observation and examination. Indeed, the sign of stupor or coma itself has diagnostic implications.

Consciousness depends on integrity of both the brainstem reticular activating system, located between the lower pons and the diencephalon, and the two cerebral hemispheres (shaded areas, Fig. 16-2). Arousal is mediated by the reticular activating system, and behavioral correlates of consciousness depend on hemispheric function. Therefore, depression of consciousness in this patient implies dysfunction of either the brainstem reticular formation or of both cerebral hemispheres.

Further refinement in the anatomic diagnosis requires more information. What do the patient's motor signs imply about corticospinal system function?

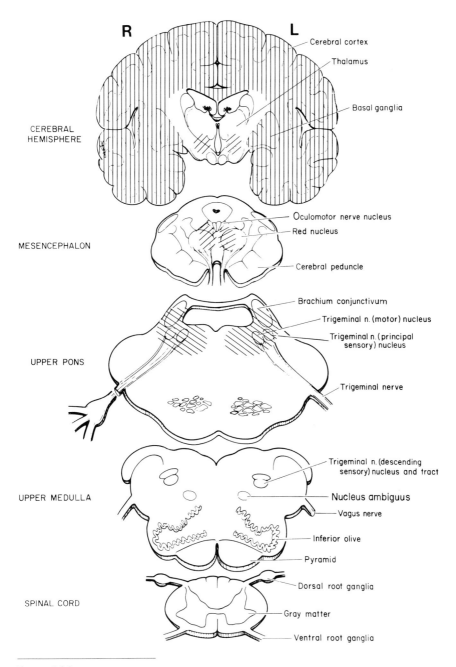

FIGURE 16-2.

Several observations in this patient imply a left-sided weakness. On the right side, but not the left, movement occurred spontaneously and in response to noxious stimuli. The left lower extremity is externally rotated, suggesting proximal leg weakness on the left. The increased muscle tone, increased reflexes, and Babinski's sign on the left side mean that the left-sided weakness is due to a lesion of the corticospinal system. Superimposing the corticospinal pathway (solid line, Fig. 16-3) on the structures involved in loss of consciousness demonstrates that the corticospinal lesion must be at or above the lower pons.

Consider the right facial weakness, as seen by the puffing out of the right cheek, flattening of the right nasolabial fold, and decreased forehead furrows on the right side. What does this imply for the anatomic diagnosis? How do the corneal reflex abnormalities aid in localizing the anatomic lesion?

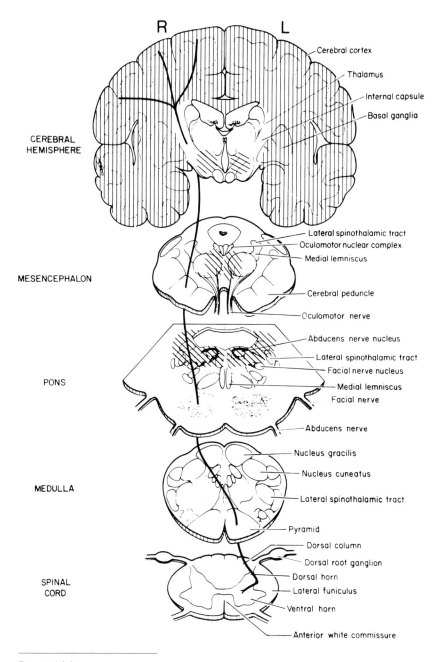

FIGURE 16-3.
Solid line: corticospinal tract.

# Case 16

The puffing out of the cheek, loss of the nasolabial fold, and decreased wrinkling on the right side of the face suggest weakness of both the upper and lower facial muscles. As seen in a previous discussion (see case 2), this weakness is most likely caused by a nuclear or peripheral facial nerve (lower motoneuron) lesion. This formulation is supported by the abnormal corneal reflexes. This reflex involves the first division of the trigeminal nerve (sensory limb) and the facial nerve (motor limb) (Fig. 16-4). If the lesion in this case affected only the trigeminal nerve, then one would expect no response of either side of the face to touching the right cornea. However, blinking of the left eye implies that sensory stimuli from the right cornea are getting into the CNS. The failure to blink on the right side is due to involvement of the motor limb of the reflex arc, hence the right facial nerve. This localization is consistent with that of the stupor and the left hemiparesis.

A pontine lesion must also explain the extraocular abnormalities elicited by the oculocephalic or doll's-head maneuver. In this case, when the head was passively rotated up, down, or to the right, the eyes moved appropriately in the opposite direction so as to maintain the initial direction of gaze. However, when the head was turned to the left, the left eye came fully to the right as expected, but the right eye moved only to the midline.

**W**hat is the mechanism underlying this abnormal response? What does this imply for the anatomic diagnosis?

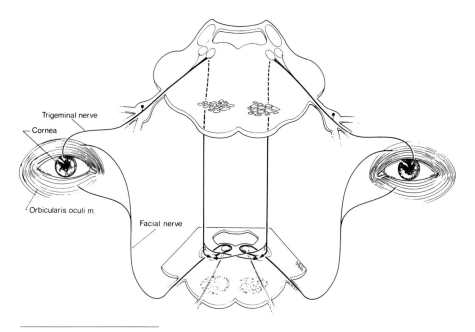

FIGURE 16-4.

## Case 16

Conjugate vertical and horizontal gaze to the left is intact, suggesting integrity of the vertical gaze centers in the midbrain and left paramedian pontine reticular formation as well as the descending supranuclear fibers to these centers (see case 2). Oculomotor, trochlear, and left abducens nerves are also intact, since the muscles supplied by these nerves are active during the oculocephalic maneuver. Although there is failure of the right eye to move to the right, the left eye is still able to do so. Therefore, the problem is not in PPRF or the abducens nerve nucleus (which would move the eyes conjugately), but in the right abducens nerve. The abducens nucleus sends fibers both to the abducens nerve and to the medial rectus subnucleus of the oculomotor complex via the medial longitudinal fasciculus located in the pons to the right of the midline. This localization is consistent with the initial hypothesis of a right pontine lesion (Fig. 16-5) affecting the corticospinal tract (solid line), right facial nerve (dotted line), and right abducens nerves (dashed line).

The location in the pons can be further refined by analyzing pontine functions that are still intact. For example, the right PPRF and abducens nucleus in the lateral pons are intact (see case 2).

What does the patient's response to pinprick mean as to sensory systems mediating pain? What does it imply for the anatomic diagnosis?

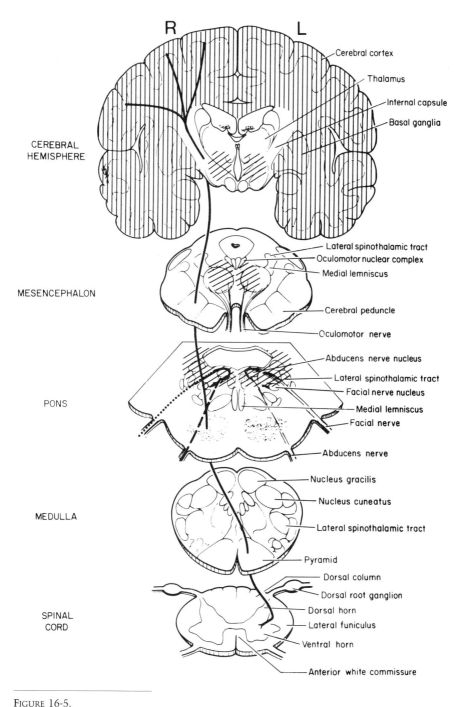

FIGURE 16-5.
Solid line: corticospinal tract; dashed line: right abducens nerve; dotted line: right facial nerve.

A response to pinprick anywhere on the body implies that the spinothalamic pathway up to and including the diencephalon is intact. However, that the patient also demonstrates a capacity to localize the pinprick on his body suggests that the spinothalamic pathway is intact all the way to the cerebral cortex (dash-dot-dash lines, Fig. 16-6). The spinothalamic pathway is lateral in the pons. This formulation is consistent with that already made of a right medial ventral pontine lesion.

The lack of other abnormal findings also supports a medial location of the lesion. A lateral pontine lesion would be expected to damage the descending nucleus of the trigeminal nerve, but the corneal reflex findings show that this is not the case. A lateral lesion might cause a Horner's syndrome from damage to the descending sympathetic fibers. Thus, this is a case of a right-sided medial pontine lesion.

There are many possibilities for the pathologic differential diagnosis. However, the sudden onset suggests a vascular cause, and the neurologic differential diagnosis would favor pontine infarction or hemorrhage. A CT scan did not show a hematoma. Therefore, the most likely neurologic diagnosis is a right medial pontine infarction due to occlusion of a penetrating branch of the basilar artery.

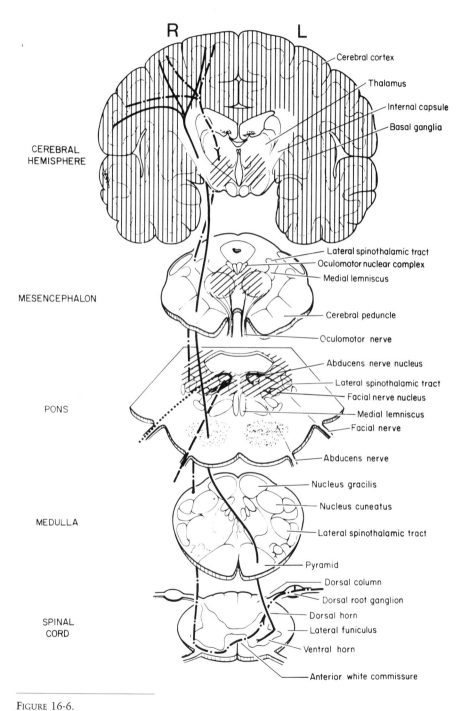

FIGURE 16-6.

Solid line: corticospinal tract; dashed line: right abducens nerve; dotted line: right facial nerve; dashed dotted line: spinothalamic tract.

**Case 17**

**Unconsciousness, Altered Respirations, and Left-Sided Weakness**

# Case 17

A 50-year-old woman with a long history of hypertension was found comatose by her nephew. The nephew stated that earlier in the day she had complained of marked headache. When he stopped by her house 2 hours later, she was lying in bed and did not respond to her name or to being shaken.

In the emergency room her blood pressure was 200/120 mm Hg. Her respirations demonstrated a waxing and waning pattern (i.e., Cheyne-Stokes respirations, Fig. 17-1). The left side of her cheek puffed out with each expiration. The patient still did not respond to her name or to being shaken. To noxious pressure above the orbit, she moved her right arm towards the stimulated site. When pinched on the right arm, she withdrew that arm; when pinched on the left, she groaned and moved her right arm slightly. No movement of the left side extremities was seen. On funduscopic examination there was disc margin elevation and blurring without venous pulsations (papilledema). The left lower extremity was externally rotated, and on that side were hypotonia, hyperreflexia, and Babinski's sign.

When the examiner held open the eyelids, the eyes were seen to be tonically deviated to the right side. Oculocephalic maneuvers failed to move the eyes from the right. After the patient's head was elevated to 30 degrees and the left external auditory canal was cleared of cerumen, the canal was slowly irrigated with ice water. Thirty seconds later both eyes moved conjugately toward the left side. There was no nystagmus. Arterial blood gases, serum electrolytes, and glucose were normal.

Analyze the patient's motor functions. What system or systems are impaired?

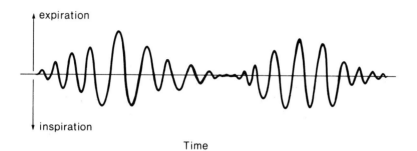

FIGURE 17-1.

## Case 17

Movement of the patient's right but not her left limbs in response to noxious stimulation, external rotation of the left lower extremity, and puffing out of the left cheek with expiration are manifestations of left-sided weakness. Left-sided hyperreflexia and Babinski's sign are further evidence that the weakness is due to a lesion of the right corticospinal pathway (solid line, Fig. 17-2). Although hypertonia is more characteristic of corticospinal pathway damage, hypotonia may be seen acutely, as in this case.

**N**ext, analyze the patient's response to noxious stimulation. What does her response imply about the pathways mediating pain sensation? How do these sensory findings contribute to the anatomic diagnosis?

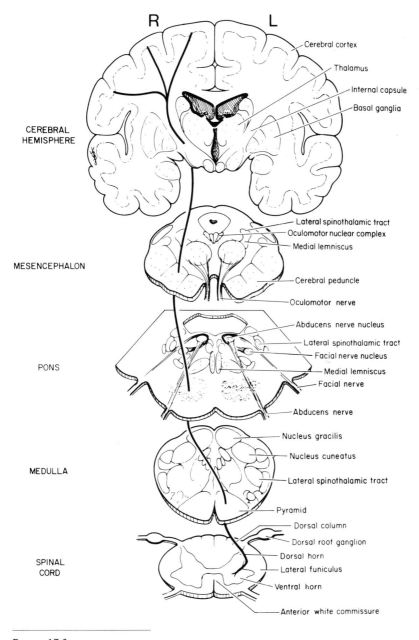

FIGURE 17-2.

Case 17

The patient's appropriate motor response to right-sided noxious stimuli, in contrast to the response to left-sided stimulation, suggests integrity of the spinothalamic pathways to the left cerebral cortex. This left sensory deficit could be caused by spinothalamic system lesions anywhere from the cutaneous receptors and peripheral nerves on the left side of the body to the right somatosensory cortex (dashed line, Fig. 17-3).

When the corticospinal, corticobulbar, and spinothalamic systems are considered together, one can see that the lesion must lie above the level of the facial nucleus in the lower pons, since there was weakness of the left side of the face, as evidenced by the left cheek puffing out with respirations. Since there was left extremity weakness, the left facial weakness would have to be due to a lesion of the corticobulbar fibers to the facial nerve. If the lesion was of the facial nucleus in the left pons, then right-sided weakness would be expected because of the lesion's involving the corticospinal tract in the left pons.

Consider the position of the eyes at rest and the response to caloric stimulation. What are the implications of these findings for the anatomic diagnosis?

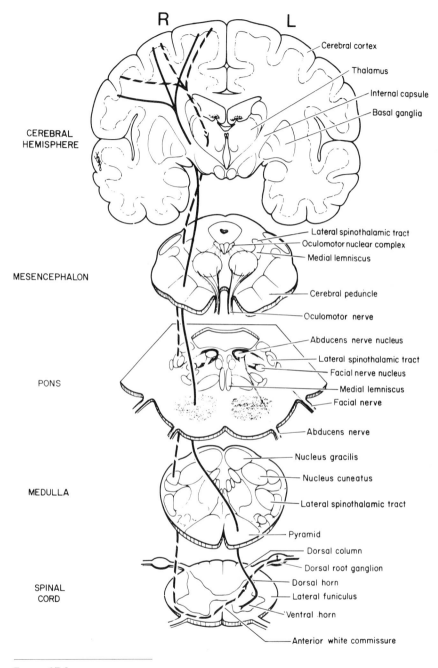

FIGURE 17-3.
Solid line: corticospinal tract; dashed line: spinothalamic tract.

## Case 17

Tonic conjugate deviation of the eyes to the right is evidence for dysfunction of mechanisms that move the eyes to the left. As described earlier (see case 2), the pathways involved in conjugate horizontal gaze to the left arise in the right cerebral hemisphere, descend through the internal capsule down the right side of the midbrain (solid line, Fig. 17-4), cross in the lower midbrain, and terminate in the left paramedian pontine reticular formation (PPRF). From there, fibers go to the left abducens nucleus. Some fibers leave the left abducens nerve, ascend in the contralateral medial longitudinal fasciculus (MLF), and synapse in the medial rectus subnucleus of the right oculomotor nuclear complex. Other fibers go with the left abducens nerve to reach the left lateral rectus muscle.

Since both eyes are affected, the lesion must involve either the right frontopontine tract above the crossing of these fibers in the lower midbrain or the left side below the lower midbrain. The latter lesion should affect adjacent corticospinal fibers causing a right, not a left, hemiparesis. Therefore, the fibers mediating left lateral gaze must be affected before they cross to the left side of the brain, and the lesion must be at or above the lower midbrain.

**A**re the findings from caloric stimulation consistent with the proposed anatomic site for the deficit of conjugate lateral gaze?

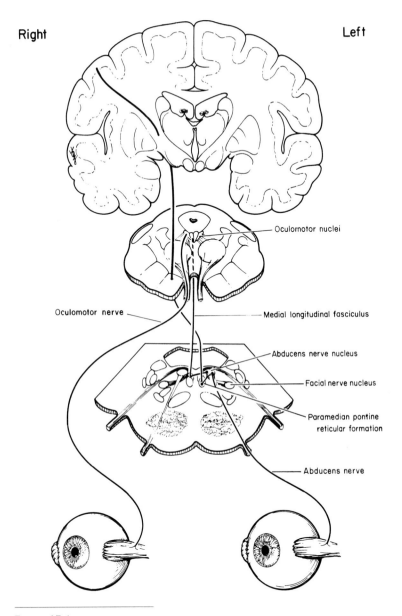

FIGURE 17-4.

Case 17

Ice water irrigation of the external auditory canal induces convection currents in the endolymphatic fluid of the labyrinths, stimulating the labyrinth. The resultant neural signal affects the vestibular nuclei and effectively stimulates the ipsilateral PPRF–abducens nuclear complex. In an awake normal person such cooling induces a lateral nystagmus whose quick phase is away from the ear being stimulated. In an unconscious patient, when the pathways described above are intact, the quick phase is lost, causing a slow tonic deviation toward the irrigated ear.

In this case, conjugate deviation of the patient's eyes to the left when the left ear was irrigated with ice water implies that the vestibular portion of the vestibulocochlear nerve, vestibular nuclei, its connections to the left PPRF abducens nucleus, MLF, and right oculomotor nucleus nuclei, and the peripheral parts of these cranial nerves are intact. Therefore, the lesion in this case lies above the midbrain and affects the supranuclear input to the PPRF (Fig. 17-5).

**W**hat do Cheyne-Stokes respirations imply as to the anatomic diagnosis?

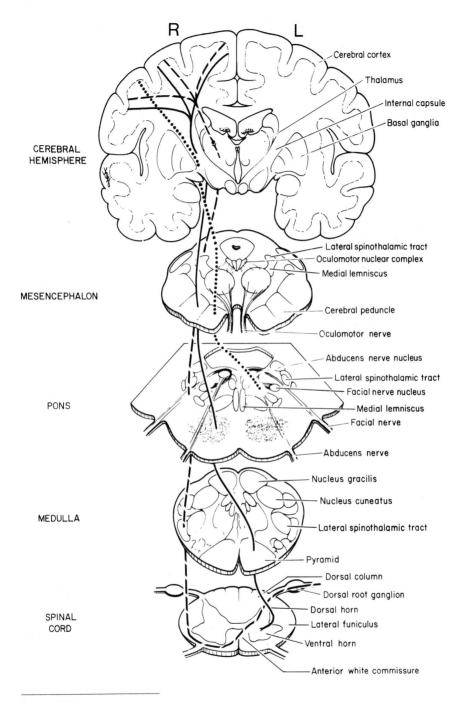

FIGURE 17-5.
Solid line: corticospinal tract; dashed line: spinothalamic tract; dotted line: frontopontine fibers to the PPRF.

Lesions in different areas of the central nervous system may be associated with specific respiratory alterations, which may have some value in anatomic localization (Fig. 17-6). However, a great deal of care is necessary, since abnormalities of the pulmonary and circulatory systems and of acid-base balance also affect respiratory patterns. Cheyne-Stokes respirations from central nervous system disease are seen with bilateral cerebral or diencephalic lesions. Apneustic breathing, a rare respiratory pattern characterized by a prolonged pause in mid-inspiration, has been associated with pontine lesions. Ataxic breathing (i.e., an irregular pattern) and respiratory arrest have been associated with medullary lesions.

In the absence of systemic metabolic derangements, Cheyne-Stokes respirations imply that a bilateral lesion involves the diencephalon or both cerebral hemispheres. The patient's motor and sensory findings suggest only a right-sided lesion of the diencephalic or cerebral hemisphere. However, some right hemisphere lesions might have some secondary effect on the other cerebral hemisphere. The neurologic differential diagnosis would favor those possibilities, since depression in the level of consciousness does not occur with damage confined to a single hemisphere.

Lesions of one cerebral hemisphere can affect the other in a variety of ways. In epilepsy, abnormal electrical activity can spread to involve the other hemisphere. Arteriovenous malformations or highly vascular tumors can shunt blood away from other parts of the brain. The most common cause, though, is increased intracranial pressure or mass effect consistent with this patient's funduscopic changes of early papilledema. Other symptoms and signs of increased intracranial pressure include headache, nausea, vomiting, visual obscurations (episodes of transient visual loss occurring in one or both eyes and lasting less than 30 seconds), horizontal diplopia from abducens nerve paresis, and papilledema.

Many disorders increase intracranial pressure by increasing the volume of the blood, brain, or CSF within the confines of the rigid skull (see case 14). Acute obstruction of cerebrospinal fluid flow (obstructive hydrocephalus) and pseudotumor cerebri (idiopathic intracranial hypertension) are associated with increased intracranial pressure, but because there is no pressure *gradient* distorting and disrupting tissue, there need not be focal findings. Edema after infarction can increase intracranial pressure, but usually does not occur until hours or several days after the initial signs of infarction. Brain tumors may cause both focal findings and increased intracranial pressure, but symptoms usually develop gradually. Rarely, a brain tumor may hemorrhage and suddenly enlarge, causing both the acute onset of focal findings and increased intracranial pressure. Intracranial hemorrhage, including subdural and epidural hematomas, ruptured aneurysms, arteriovenous malformation, and hypertensive hemorrhages, similarly produces sudden focal findings superimposed on signs of increased intracranial pressure. Subdural and epidural hematomas usually follow trauma to the head.

In this case CT scan demonstrated an intracerebral hemorrhage deep within the right hemisphere.

*CHEYNE-STOKES*

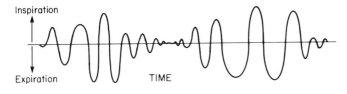

*APNEUSTIC*

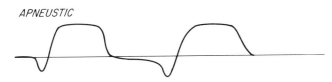

*ATAXIC RESPIRATION*

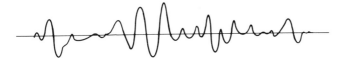

FIGURE 17-6.

**Case 18**

# Unconsciousness

## Case 18

A 19-year-old woman was found lying in her hospital bed unresponsive. Six days previously she had been admitted to the hospital for abdominal pain. No explanation for the abdominal pain had been discovered, and she was being readied for discharge. The patient had received no medications except for a minor tranquilizer the previous day.

The patient was lying supine in bed. Blood pressure, pulse, and respirations were normal. She did not respond to her name or to gentle shaking. When the eyelids were passively opened, both eyes were positioned upward and outward (Fig. 18-1). After a few seconds the eyes moved to direct forward gaze. The pupils were 3 mm in diameter and reacted normally to light. With oculocephalic (doll's-head) maneuvers the eyes maintained their straight-ahead position relative to the head. The eyelids closed quickly when released. The nasolabial folds were symmetric, and gag and corneal reflexes were intact. There was no response to noxious stimuli, including pinprick, the pinching of the Achilles' tendon, or pressure to the fingernail beds. Muscle tone was normal. When either arm was lifted directly over the face and released, it fell laterally, thereby avoiding striking the face. Tendon reflexes were normal and Babinski's sign was absent. Irrigation of the right external auditory canal with ice water caused a left-beating horizontal nystagmus. Arterial blood gas and serum electrolytes and glucose values were normal.

What is the nature of the patient's weakness? Where is the anatomic lesion that would explain the motor findings?

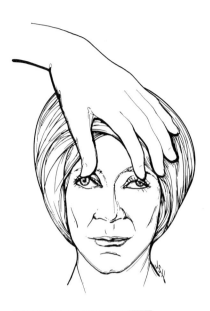

FIGURE 18-1.

Failure of the limbs and face to move spontaneously or in response to noxious stimuli may suggest generalized weakness or a severe depression of consciousness. Weakness may be caused by lesions affecting the upper motoneuron, lower motoneuron, peripheral nerve, neuromuscular junction, or muscle. The absence of hyperreflexia, hypertonia, and Babinski's sign suggests that an upper motoneuron lesion is unlikely. The absence of hypotonia and hyporeflexia suggests that a peripheral nerve or lower motoneuron lesion is unlikely. The remaining possibilities include disorders of the neuromuscular junction and muscle. However, these possibilities, as well as those of the peripheral nerve and lower motoneuron, are inconsistent with the patient's decreased level of consciousness, which implies a CNS lesion at or above the lower pons or metabolic encephalopathy.

Closer review of the physical examination reveals that the patient is not truly without any motor function. During the examination her arm was held above her face such that when released it would have struck the face had it fallen freely. However, her arm fell to the side, avoiding the face. This finding implies that the patient moved the arm to the side, and, what is more important, that she recognized the need to do so. This response is inconsistent with her failure to respond to other stimuli. At this point a conversion reaction or malingering must be considered. Is there other evidence to support this possibility? What do the extraocular muscle function and her response to ice water caloric testing suggest regarding the functional integrity of the systems controlling eye movement?

When the eyelids were first opened, the eyes were positioned up and out. This is the normal Bell's phenomenon. Nystagmus during ice water calorics is also a normal response in a conscious person. Patients with intact ocular motility systems but decreased level of consciousness usually do not have nystagmus. Rather, the eyes drift slowly toward the side irrigated with cold water. In patients with a decreased level of consciousness, the eyelids usually drift down slowly when released. In this patient the eyelids quickly closed. All these findings support the diagnosis of a conversion reaction or malingering.

The diagnosis of a conversion reaction or malingering depends on the clinical findings. It is not a diagnosis of exclusion. It depends on eliciting symptoms and signs that are inconsistent with anatomic or physiologic fact. For example, loss of sensation that stops exactly in the midline would be extremely unusual for a lesion of the sensory systems. Vibration on one side of the forehead near the midline or sternum is transmitted bilaterally by bone conduction. As such, vibratory sensation should be perceived on both sides of the forehead or sternum regardless of which side is stimulated, even in the presence of a unilateral organic sensory impairment.

Patients with factitious anosmia may state that they do not smell any odor, including ammonia. However, ammonia irritates the nasal mucosa, a sensation that is mediated by the trigeminal, not the olfactory, nerve. Occasional unsophisticated patients may complain of decreased sensation in one leg while supine. When turned prone, they may then complain of decreased sensation in the other leg.

In testing for Romberg's sign in patients with factitious ataxia, the center of gravity remains over the feet despite wild gyrations of the hips and trunk. A supine patient with functional low back pain may report pain as the hip is flexed with the knee extended (a positive straight leg raising test). However, at other times the patient may uncomplainingly sit with hips fully flexed and knees fully extended.

The finding of Hoover's sign suggests that a patient is not making a maximal effort to flex the hip of an allegedly weak lower extremity. Hoover's sign is the failure to exert downward force (i.e., hip extension) of the other, presumably intact, leg sufficient to permit flexion of the affected leg at the hip. Hoover's sign would thus support the impression of functional leg weakness.

The patient in this case abruptly and spontaneously recovered later the same day. Samples of blood and urine, obtained while she was unresponsive, confirmed the absence of drugs or toxins. She offered no explanation and denied that she had voluntarily produced the unresponsiveness. In the absence of evidence to support volitional control of the symptoms and signs, this episode might represent a conversion reaction. Subsequent psychiatric evaluation suggested that the presence of an intolerable domestic situation may have been etiologically important in her symptoms.

# Case 19

## Unresponsiveness and Ophthalmoplegia

## Case 19

A 42-year-old construction worker with a history of high blood pressure suddenly slumped to the ground. According to his foreman, he had complained bitterly of right-sided head pain and double vision just a short time before. His speech was slurred, and he had some difficulty in lifting his left arm. Half an hour later, paramedics reported that he was difficult to arouse and was unable to move his left limbs.

In the hospital his blood pressure was 240/125 mm Hg. The patient lay quietly with his eyes closed. He responded to noxious stimuli by opening his eyes, grimacing, and using his right limbs to ward off the examiner. On his left side, there was an extensor (decerebrate) response (Fig. 19-1A) to painful stimuli. When the eyelids were lifted, his right eye was seen to deviate down and laterally, and his left eye deviated medially (Fig. 19-1B). Spontaneously or with oculocephalic (doll's-head) maneuvers, the right eye abducted fully, but it would not move in any other direction. The left eye had full movements except for a failure of abduction, which could not be overcome by the oculocephalic maneuver. The left pupil was 3 mm in diameter and reacted normally. On spontaneous downward gaze the right eye rotated in a clockwise direction (intorsion). The right pupil was 7 mm in diameter and did not react to light. Bilateral papilledema was present. When he grimaced to noxious stimulation, the muscles of facial expression were weak in the lower portion of the left face. Present on the left were hyperactive tendon reflexes and Babinski's sign.

Where is the lesion that would cause the patient's symptoms and signs? Consider first his motor disturbance.

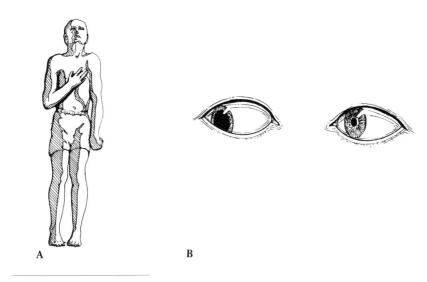

FIGURE 19-1.

## Case 19

Left-sided weakness, extensor (decerebrate) response, hyperreflexia, and Babinski's sign implicate a lesion of corticospinal and corticobulbar fibers arising from the right cerebral hemisphere. The lesion must be rostral to the lower pons because facial weakness is present.

Although the left hemiparesis is consistent with a right hemispheric lesion, the decreased level of consciousness is not. Either both hemispheres or the brainstem must also be involved. These other areas may be involved indirectly by mass effect, where an enlarging lesion of one hemisphere may compress the other hemisphere or brainstem. An expanding lesion would also cause increased intracranial pressure, as evidenced by the presence of papilledema on funduscopic examination. However, any anatomic diagnosis must also explain the patient's oculomotor findings.

Figure 19-2 shows the activities of each of the extraocular muscles in moving the eyes. The lateral recti, which abduct the eyes, are innervated by the abducens nerves. The medial recti adduct the eyes and are innervated by the oculomotor nerves. The oculomotor nerves also innervate the inferior and superior recti, which move the eyes downward and upward, respectively. The inferior oblique muscles, also innervated by the oculomotor nerves, move the eyes upward and extort them. The superior oblique, innervated by the trochlear nerve, moves the eyes downward and intorts them.

**W**here is the lesion that would produce this patient's deficits of ocular motility and his pupillary abnormalities?

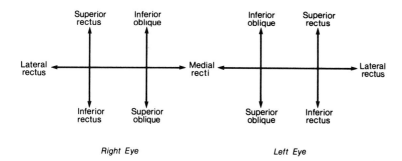

FIGURE 19-2.

The medial, superior, and inferior recti and inferior oblique are paralyzed in the right eye. These extraocular muscles are innervated by the oculomotor nerve. The conclusion, then, is a lesion of the right oculomotor nerve. (Recall from case 8 that fibers to the right superior rectus arise from the left oculomotor nucleus. Therefore, this patient's lesion cannot be nuclear.) The clockwise rotatory motion (intorsion) present on down gaze implies that the fourth nerve is functioning (it is primarily an intorter and depressor). The left eye cannot abduct, implying a lateral rectus or abducens nerve lesion. How is it possible for a single lesion to affect both the right oculomotor nerve and left abducens nerve? Could this abduction deficit be explained as being part of a supranuclear conjugate gaze palsy to the right?

Trace out the pathways for the control of voluntary gaze. Remember that the pathway originates in the frontal eye fields, descends in the internal capsule and cerebral peduncles, crosses just below the level of the trochlear nucleus, and synapses in the paramedian pontine reticular formation (PPRF) (Fig. 19-3). The PPRF activates the abducens nerve nucleus and its two populations of neurons, that is, motoneurons to the ipsilateral lateral rectus and internuclear neurons, which cross in the lower pons and ascend in the medial longitudinal fasciculus to reach the contralateral medial rectus subnucleus of the oculomotor nerve. Motoneurons leave the medial rectus subnucleus to innervate the medial rectus.

The oculocephalic maneuver, in which the patient's head is briskly turned and the patient's eye movements are observed, tests the vestibuloocular reflex, which produces an equal but opposite eye movement to each head movement, thus maintaining fixation. The vestibuloocular pathway originates in the semicircular canals. A synapse occurs in the vestibular nucleus, and fibers then pass up the brainstem to each of the three ocular motor nuclei. The oculocephalic maneuver in a comatose patient with an intact eye movement system causes full and conjugate horizontal and vertical eye movements. Ice water irrigation in a comatose patient with an intact vestibuloocular eye movement system produces tonic conjugate deviation of the eyes toward the irrigated side.

Supranuclear conjugate gaze palsies, therefore, can be overcome by the oculocephalic maneuver or ice water caloric irrigation; but lesions of the nuclei, internuclear connections, and oculomotor, trochlear, and abducens nerves cannot. The last was the case in this patient: There was paralysis of the right oculomotor nerve and the left abducens.

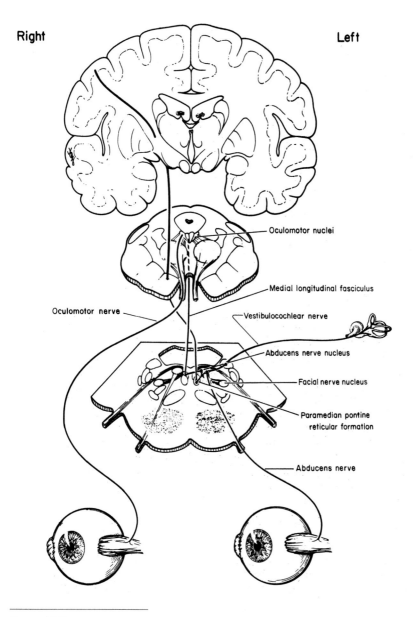

FIGURE 19-3.

The lesion cannot be localized to one discrete area of the central nervous system. The right oculomotor nerve and left abducens nerve are not in close proximity either in or near the brainstem as indicated by analysis of the previous findings. An empiric observation important in neurologic diagnosis is that abducens nerve palsies may occur in the setting of increased intracranial pressure. This is an indirect effect called a false localizing sign, since it may give the erroneous impression of a brainstem lesion.

The anatomic diagnosis to this point of analysis is a lesion of the right cerebral hemisphere, which is producing increased intracranial pressure. The right oculomotor nerve palsy has yet to be explained. Does the proposed anatomic lesion explain the right third nerve palsy?

With increased intracranial pressure there may be pressure gradients that may cause tissue to shift or move from a region of high pressure to one of lower pressure. This shifting can disrupt tissue or its blood supply. The intracranial contents are divided by dural sheaths including the falx cerebri and the tentorium cerebelli. These dural sheaths partition the brain into three compartments, the right and left supratentorial compartments and the infratentorial compartment. When there is an expanding mass in one compartment, tissue may shift (herniate) into another compartment of lower pressure. Certain anatomic locations are affected, thus giving rise to specific symptoms and signs. Brain contents may also herniate through the foramen magnum.

Cingulate herniation (Fig. 19-4C) is due to an expanding hemispheric mass, which causes shift of the cingulate gyrus under the falx cerebri. The herniated tissue may compress the anterior cerebral artery, resulting in infarction of the medial convexity of the hemisphere, causing contralateral lower extremity weakness.

Central transtentorial herniation occurs when medially placed expanding supratentorial lesions caudally displace the diencephalon and the adjoining midbrain through the tentorial notch (Fig. 19-4B). The initial sign of lethargy is followed by signs of diencephalic dysfunction (i.e., Cheyne-Stokes respirations, small reactive pupils, and Babinski's sign). With continued expansion of the mass, the patient lapses into coma. Next, signs of midbrain and upper pontine dysfunction develop. The vestibuloocular reflexes are lost, the pupils become midposition and fixed to light, and a flaccid quadraparesis or decerebrate posturing results. The respiratory pattern may be that of central neurogenic hyperventilation or apneustic breathing (case 17). In the latter, lower pontine–upper medulla stage breathing may become slow and irregular. Pulse and blood pressure are maintained, but no other evidence of brainstem function is present.

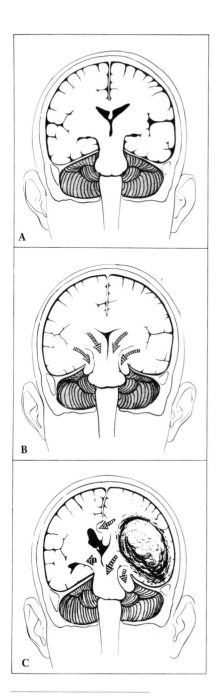

FIGURE 19-4.
Reproduced with permission from Plum, F., and Posner, J. *The Diagnosis of Stupor and Coma* (3rd ed.). Philadelphia: Davis, 1980.

When masses in the lateral portion of the hemispheres or temporal lobe expand, the uncus of the temporal lobe herniates through a notch in the tentorium cerebelli (uncal herniation, Fig. 19-4C). Dilatation and sluggish light reflex of the pupil on the side of the expanding mass, are due to oculomotor nerve compression. Later, the posterior cerebral artery may be compromised, causing a homonymous hemianopsia. The patient discussed in this case had signs of uncal herniation.

This stage is followed by a complete oculomotor nerve palsy on the side of the expanding mass. The oculomotor nerve courses near the free edge of the tentorial notch and is vulnerable to early compression by the herniating uncus. With further herniation, the ipsilateral midbrain is compressed, causing decerebration. Further compression causes the same picture as seen in the midbrain–upper pontine stage and later the lower pontine–upper medullary stage described above.

Two herniation syndromes are associated with expanding lesions in the posterior fossa. Upward transtentorial herniation occurs when the mesencephalon and cerebellum herniate superiorly through the tentorial notch (Fig. 19-5A). There are signs of the inciting brainstem involvement, often with symmetrically miotic pupils. Compression of the oculomotor nerves and mesencephalon by the upwardly shifting tissue results in pupillary dilatation (sometimes unequally) to midposition and loss of the pupillary light reaction. Compression of the rostral midbrain may cause vertical gaze deficits and decerebration.

The final herniation syndrome occurs when the cerebellar tonsils are forced through the foramen magnum (Fig. 19-5B). Initially, the patient may complain of a stiff neck. The ensuing compression of the medulla and upper spinal cord leads to circulatory collapse, respiratory arrest, and death.

The pathologic differential diagnosis of a unilateral hemispheric lesion has been covered previously. Which of these possibilities are expanding mass lesions? Which are most likely? The neurologic differential diagnosis would include (1) intraparenchymal hemorrhage, (2) subdural hematoma, (3) primary or metastatic tumor with hemorrhage into it, (4) brain abscess, and (5) epidural hematoma, since there was sudden onset of symptoms suggesting a vascular cause as well as evidence of an expanding mass lesion.

Intraparenchymal hemorrhages are common in hypertensive patients but also occur from trauma, ruptured aneurysms, and arteriovenous malformations. A CT scan showed a large high-attenuation (i.e., dense) mass in the basal ganglia and corona radiata of the right hemisphere with compression of the right cerebral peduncle. Thus, the neurologic diagnosis is hypertensive intracerebral hemorrhage with uncal herniation and abducens nerve paresis secondary to increased intracranial pressure.

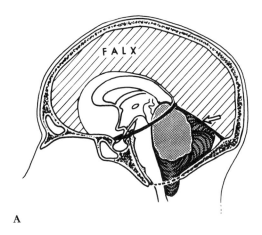

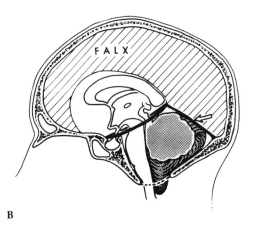

FIGURE 19-5.
Reproduced with permission from Cuneo, R., et al. Upward transtentorial herniation. *Arch. Neurol.* 36:619, 1979. Copyright 1979, American Medical Association.

**Case 20**

# Weakness and Sensory Loss in the Right Hand

## Case 20

Over the previous 4 months a 42-year-old right-handed school teacher noted the gradual inability to perform fine motor tasks with his right hand and a tingling sensation involving the right ring and little fingers. He also noticed wasting between the base of his thumb and index finger. Buttoning his shirts and writing became difficult. There was no weakness, numbness, or tingling of his other extremities. He was an intense man who spent much of his time, both in school and at home, seated at his desk reading or correcting papers.

Cranial nerve functions were normal. The right thumb, index, and middle fingers were extended, the ring finger was slightly flexed, and the little finger was moderately flexed. There was extension of the fingers at the metacarpophalangeal joints, and the hand was deviated toward the radial side of the arm. (This posture is that of the claw hand deformity, Fig. 20-1.) There were wasting and fasciculations of the right hypothenar eminence. Adduction and opposition of the little finger, adduction and abduction of the index finger, and thumb adduction were weak. The remainder of movements in the right upper extremity were of normal strength. Muscle strength and bulk were normal in the left upper extremity and the lower extremities.

Pain, temperature, and touch sensation were diminished in the little finger, the medial half of the ring finger, and the medial one-third of the hand, affecting both the palmar and dorsal surfaces (Fig. 20-1). Sensory symptoms could be easily reproduced by gently tapping behind the right medial epicondyle with a reflex hammer. On the left side, however, the tap required to produce similar paresthesias in the left hand was much stronger than on the right. Coordination, gait, and tendon reflexes were normal, and Babinski's signs were absent.

Is the patient's weakness due to a lesion of the upper motoneuron, lower motoneuron, peripheral nerve, neuromuscular junction, or muscle?

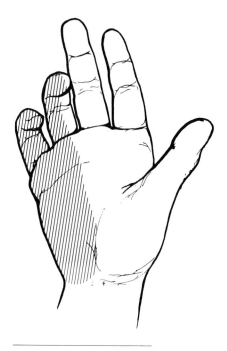

FIGURE 20-1.

## Case 20

Lesions of upper motoneurons cause weakness with increased tone, hyperreflexia, and Babinski's signs, whereas lower motoneuron (anterior horn cell) lesions cause weakness with muscle wasting, hypotonia, fasciculations, and reflex loss. Peripheral nerve lesions cause muscle wasting, hypotonia, reflex loss, and sensory loss, most often without fasciculations. Lesions of the neuromuscular junction and muscle cause weakness without fasciculations or changes in reflexes (Table 20-1).

This patient's sensory loss is not consistent with a lesion of the anterior horn cell, neuromuscular junction, or muscle. Disease of the neuromuscular junction is characterized by weakness that worsens with exercise (for example, the fatigability of myasthenia gravis). Myopathies are usually characterized by proximal muscle weakness in all extremities.

Because of focal weakness, wasting, and sensory loss, this patient's findings are best explained by a lesion of the peripheral nerve. Which peripheral nerve is involved and where along its course is the lesion?

Table 20-1.
Clinical findings associated with lesions at various levels of the motor system

| | Upper Motoneuron | Anterior Horn Cell | Peripheral Nerve | Neuromuscular Junction | Muscle |
|---|---|---|---|---|---|
| Pattern of weakness | Unilateral or bilateral | Generalized or localized | Depends on nerve(s) involved | Most often generalized | Proximal greater than distal |
| Reflexes | Increased | Decreased | Decreased if reflex arc is affected by the lesion | Normal until weakness is severe; then decreased | Normal until weakness is severe; then decreased |
| Wasting | Mild | Marked | Moderate to marked | Mild | Mild |
| Fasciculations | Absent | Marked | Absent or rare | Absent | Absent |
| Sensory loss | Absent | Absent | Common; depends on nerve(s) involved | Absent | Absent |

**Case 20**

The peripheral nerves of the upper extremities can be diagrammed as in Figure 20-2. As the nerves exit the spinal cord, they form the dorsal and ventral roots, which exit through the neural foramina of the vertebral column and combine to form the upper, middle, and lower trunks of the brachial plexus. Each trunk bifurcates into an anterior and posterior division, and these divisions unite to form the lateral, medial, and posterior cords of the brachial plexus. The cords then divide into nerves, which branch to the muscles and sensory receptors of the upper extremities. Where in this system could a lesion explain the patient's symptoms and signs? (Table 20-2 may be used.) Note that the following muscles of the right upper extremity are weak:

1. Flexor carpi ulnaris
2. Flexor digitorum profundus (ring and little fingers)
3. Abductor digiti minimi
4. Opponens digiti minimi
5. Flexor digiti minimi
6. Dorsal interossei
7. Palmar interossei
8. Adductor pollicis

As seen in Table 20-2, all of these muscles are innervated by the C8, T1 roots, the lower trunk of the brachial plexus, anterior division, and the medial cords of the brachial plexus and the ulnar nerve. It is now necessary to determine which of these five sites is the locus of the lesion.

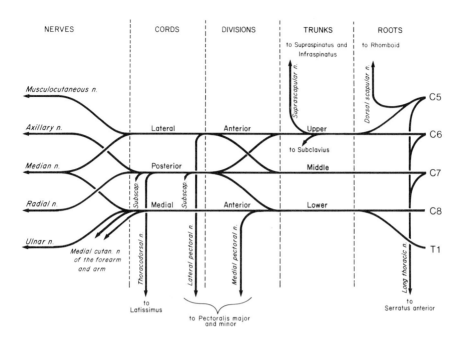

FIGURE 20-2.

Table 20-2.
Muscles of the upper extremity, their associated roots, trunks, divisions, cords, and peripheral nerves

| Muscle | Root | Trunk |
|---|---|---|
| Rhomboids | C4–C5 | |
| Pectoralis major | C5–C6 | Upper |
| | C7 | Middle |
| | C8–T1 | Lower |
| Supraspinatus | C5 | Upper |
| Infraspinatus | C5–C6 | Upper |
| Latissimus dorsi | C6 | Upper |
| | C7 | Middle |
| | C8 | Lower |
| Biceps | C5–C6 | Upper |
| Deltoid | C5–C6 | Upper |
| Triceps | C7 | Middle |
| | C8 | Lower |
| Brachioradialis | C5–C6 | Upper |
| Extensor carpi radialis longus | C6 | Upper |
| | C7 | Middle |
| Supinator | C5–C6 | Upper |
| Extensor digitorum | C7 | Middle |
| | C8 | Lower |
| Extensor carpi ulnaris | C7 | Middle |
| | C8 | Lower |
| Abductor pollicis longus | C7 | Middle |
| | C8 | Lower |
| Extensor pollicis brevis | C7 | Middle |
| | C8 | Lower |
| Extensor pollicis longus | C7 | Middle |
| | C8 | Lower |
| Pronator teres | C6 | Upper |
| | C7 | Middle |
| Flexor carpi radialis | C6 | Upper |
| | C7 | Middle |
| Flexor digitorum sublimis | C8 | Lower |
| | C8–T1 | Middle |
| | C7 | Lower |
| Flexor digitorum profundus I, II | C8–T1 | Lower |
| Flexor pollicis longus | C8–T1 | Lower |
| Abductor pollicis brevis | C8–T1 | Lower |
| Opponens pollicis | C8–T1 | Lower |
| 1st and 2nd lumbrical and interosseous muscles | C8–T1 | Lower |
| Flexor carpi ulnaris | C8 | Lower |
| Flexor digitorum profundus III, IV | C8–T1 | Lower |
| Abductor digiti minimi | C8–T1 | Lower |
| First dorsal interosseous | C8–T1 | Lower |
| First palmar interosseous | C8–T1 | Lower |
| Adductor pollicis | C8–T1 | Lower |
| Opponens digiti minimi | C8–T1 | Lower |

Used with permission from E. R. Seringa. In P. G. Vinken and G. W. Bruyn. *Handbook of Clinical Neurology.* Amsterdam: Elsevier, 1969. Vol. 2. Pp. 132–133.

| Division | Cord | Peripheral Nerve |
|---|---|---|
| | | Dorsal scapular nerve |
| Anterior | | Lateral pectoral nerve |
| Anterior | | Lateral pectoral nerve |
| Anterior | Medial | Medial pectoral nerve |
| | | Suprascapular nerve |
| | | Suprascapular nerve |
| Posterior | Posterior | Thoracodorsal nerve |
| Posterior | Posterior | Thoracodorsal nerve |
| Posterior | Posterior | Thoracodorsal nerve |
| Anterior | Lateral | Musculocutaneous nerve |
| Posterior | Posterior | Axillary nerve |
| Posterior | Posterior | Radial nerve |
| Posterior | Posterior | Radial nerve |
| Posterior | Posterior | Radial nerve |
| Posterior | Posterior | Radial nerve |
| Posterior | Posterior | Radial nerve |
| Posterior | Posterior | Radial nerve |
| Posterior | Posterior | Radial nerve |
| Posterior | Posterior | Radial nerve |
| Posterior | Posterior | Radial nerve |
| Posterior | Posterior | Radial nerve |
| Posterior | Posterior | Radial nerve |
| Posterior | Posterior | Radial nerve |
| Posterior | Posterior | Radial nerve |
| Posterior | Posterior | Radial nerve |
| Posterior | Posterior | Radial nerve |
| Posterior | Posterior | Radial nerve |
| Anterior | Lateral | Median nerve |
| Anterior | Lateral | Median nerve |
| Anterior | Lateral | Median nerve |
| Anterior | Lateral | Median nerve |
| Anterior | Lateral | Median nerve |
| Anterior | Medial | Median nerve |
| Anterior | Medial | Median nerve |
| Anterior | Medial | Median nerve |
| Anterior | Medial | Median nerve |
| Anterior | Medial | Median nerve |
| Anterior | Medial | Median nerve |
| Anterior | Medial | Median and ulnar nerves |
| Anterior | Medial | Ulnar nerve |
| Anterior | Medial | Ulnar nerve |
| Anterior | Medial | Ulnar nerve |
| Anterior | Medial | Ulnar nerve |
| Anterior | Medial | Ulnar nerve |
| Anterior | Medial | Ulnar nerve |
| Anterior | Medial | Ulnar nerve |

Lesions of the T1 nerve root cause weakness and wasting of the intrinsic hand muscles. The only two intrinsic hand muscles that do not receive some innervation from the ulnar nerve are the opponens pollicis and abductor pollicis brevis (both median nerve innervated). Since these muscles are spared and are innervated by the T1 nerve root, the patient does not have a root lesion.

The lower trunk supplies not only the muscles involved in our case but many others, such as the pectoralis major, latissimus dorsi, triceps, extensor carpi ulnaris, abductor pollicis, and extensor digitorum. Similarly, one can deduce from Table 20-2 that the anterior division and medial cord supply the pectoralis major, flexor digitorum sublimus, flexor pollicis longus, abductor pollicis brevis, and opponens pollicis, all of which are normal in this patient. The conclusion is that a right ulnar nerve lesion is responsible for the patient's symptoms and signs.

The ulnar nerve may be affected anywhere along its course. Review which muscles are affected. The ulnar nerve must be affected proximal to the branches to the involved muscles (Fig. 20-3).

All muscles innervated by the ulnar nerve are affected. The branch to the flexor carpi ulnaris is the most proximal branch affected. Its takeoff is just distal to the elbow. The lesion is, therefore, distal to the brachial plexus yet proximal to the branch to the flexor carpi ulnaris.

In this case nerve conduction studies confirmed a conduction block at the elbow. The ulnar nerve at the elbow is particularly liable to injury. Behind the medial epicondyle it is just beneath the skin, but elsewhere it is better protected by bone and soft tissue.

Other nerves are vulnerable at certain anatomic sites. The median nerve is commonly entrapped at the wrist between the carpal bones and the flexor retinaculum, causing symptoms of the carpal tunnel syndrome. The radial nerve is susceptible to pressure against the medial aspect of the upper arm, causing a wrist drop. This is sometimes referred to as the Saturday night palsy, since it often occurs when a person drops an arm over the back of a chair or bench after a long evening of imbibing alcohol. The common peroneal nerve is susceptible to compression as it passes laterally over the head of the fibula. Prolonged leg crossing or high top boots can thus cause a foot drop.

This patient reported that he spends much time at his desk writing. When one observed him at this task, it could be seen that he presses down hard with his right forearm and elbow. In fact, he stated that he had modified his writing style because of mild pain in his elbow as he writes. Treatment for this patient consisted of modification of his writing style so that there was no longer compression of the ulnar nerve at the elbow. Over the following year his symptoms and signs gradually resolved.

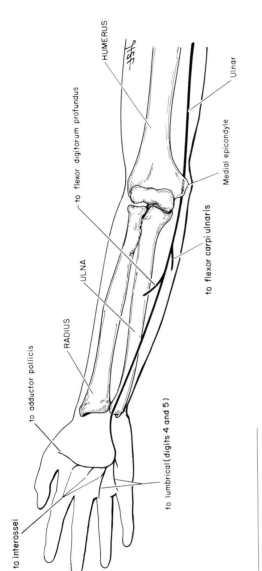

FIGURE 20-3.

**Case 21**

# Traumatic Weakness and Numbness of the Right Arm, with Anisocoria

# Case 21

A 19-year-old student was hospitalized after a motorcycle accident. He never lost consciousness, but he was unable to move his right hand following the accident, and he had sustained other severe injuries. A month later he sought outpatient evaluation for persistent weakness and numbness of his right arm and hand.

Although it was difficult for him to move the fingers and thumb of his right hand, upper and lower extremity strength was otherwise normal. He remarked that the ring and little finger of his right hand and the medial side of his hand, forearm, and arm had consistently felt "dead" or "numb" to the touch.

The vital signs were normal, and he was alert and oriented. Speech was normal. The skin of the right forehead was smoother to the touch than on the left. The right eyelid drooped (the right palpebral fissure width was 4 mm and the left was 7), and pupil diameters differed (the right was 2 mm and the left was 4). Other cranial nerve functions were normal. There was striking loss of muscle bulk of the right thenar and hypothenar eminences. Due to interossei wasting, the metacarpals were prominent beneath the skin on the dorsal aspect of this hand. Associated with this muscle wasting was marked weakness principally affecting individual muscles of the right hand (Table 21-1). Over the ring and little fingers, along the medial aspect of the right forearm and arm, and extending to include the posterior thorax, sensation was impaired for all the modalities tested (pinprick, light touch with a wisp of cotton, pressure, passive movements of the fourth and fifth digits, and a vibrating tuning fork) (Fig. 21-1). Tendon reflexes, coordination, and gait were normal.

Is the weakness of the right hand caused by dysfunction at the level of the upper motoneuron, anterior horn cell, peripheral nerve, neuromuscular junction, or muscle?

Table 21-1.
Right upper extremity motor functions involved in this case and their responsible muscles

| Motor function | Weak muscle(s) | Strength* |
|---|---|---|
| Elbow extension | Triceps | 4 |
| Wrist flexion | Flexor carpi radialis and ulnaris | 4 |
| Wrist extension | Extensor carpi radialis and ulnaris | 4 |
| Finger flexion | Flexor digitorum profundus and sublimis | 1 |
| Index finger abduction | First dorsal interosseus | 0 |
| Thumb extension | Extensor pollicis longus and brevis | 4 |
| Thumb abduction | Abductor pollicis brevis | 0 |
| Thumb adduction | Adductor pollicis | 0 |
| Thumb opposition | Opponens pollicis | 0 |

* Grades of muscle strength: 0 = no contraction; 1 = contraction of muscle but no movement of joint; 2 = movement of joint but not against gravity; 3 = movement against gravity but without any additional resistance; 4 = movement against added resistence but still weak; and 5 = normal strength.

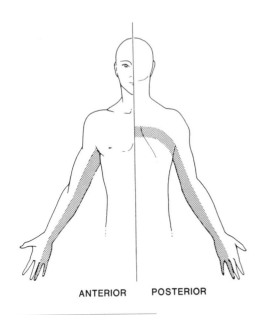

ANTERIOR    POSTERIOR

FIGURE 21-1.

The absence of such signs as hyperreflexia and hypertonia implies that there is no involvement of the corticospinal system. Muscle wasting from disuse or possibly from a lack of nerve-dependent trophic factors for the muscle fibers is the hallmark of muscle denervation from anterior horn cell (lower motoneuron) disease or peripheral nerve sectioning. Although lesser degrees of wasting also follow disuse from other causes (myopathy, myasthenia gravis, prolonged bed rest, etc.), the striking atrophy in this case makes these possibilities unlikely. His associated sensory loss similarly excludes primary involvement of anterior horn cells, the neuromuscular junction, and the muscle itself. Most nerves contain motor and sensory axons, and both weakness and numbness follow peripheral nerve damage. This patient's weakness is, therefore, due to damage within the peripheral nervous system.

In the upper extremity, nerve damage might occur to roots as they exit the spinal cord, to the brachial plexus where root fibers intermingle, or to individual peripheral nerves formed from the plexus (Fig. 21-2). Are the findings those of root, plexus, or peripheral nerve injury?

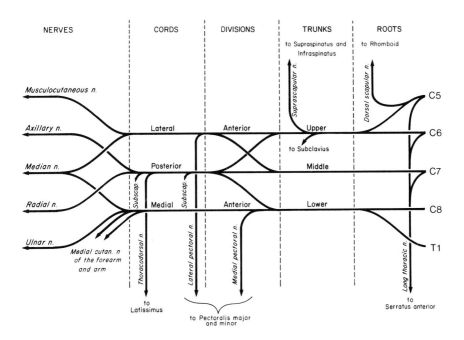

FIGURE 21-2.

## Case 21

All the weak muscles in this patient are innervated from C8 and T1 nerve roots (Table 21-2). Involvement of the triceps and extensor carpi ulnaris and radialis might suggest radial nerve damage. However, normal function of the brachioradialis, which is also innervated by the radial nerve, precludes involvement of this nerve. Median or ulnar nerve lesions would not explain the weakness of the triceps and the extensor carpi radialis and ulnaris. Similar analysis of the brachial plexus projections to the involved muscles also excludes involvement of either the divisions or cords of the brachial plexus. However, damage to the lower trunk of the right brachial plexus or C8 and T1 nerve roots would explain this patient's pattern of muscle weakness. The pattern of sensory loss (see Fig. 21-1) is that of C8 and T1 dermatomes (Fig. 21-3), supporting an anatomic diagnosis of either the lower trunk of the right brachial plexus or the right C8 and T1 nerve roots.

What are implications of the patient's anisocoria and right ptosis? Is the anisocoria caused by an afferent (sensory) or efferent (motor) deficit?

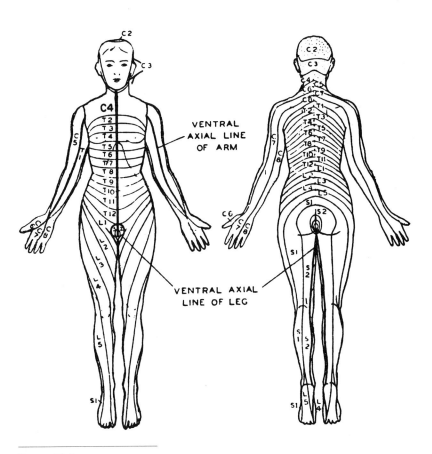

Figure 21-3.

Table 21-2.
Some of the Muscles of the Upper Extremities, Their Innervation by Peripheral Nerves and Nerve Roots

| Muscle | Plexus | Peripheral Nerves | | |
|---|---|---|---|---|
| | | Ulnar | Median | Radial |
| Supraspinatus | X | | | |
| Deltoid | | | | |
| Biceps | | | | |
| Brachioradialis | | | | X |
| Triceps* | | | | X |
| Flexor carpi radialis | | | X | |
| Flexor carpi ulnaris* | | | | X |
| Extensor carpi radialis and | | | | X |
| ulnaris* | | | | X |
| Supinator | | | | X |
| Pronator teres | | | X | |
| Extensor digitorum* | | | | X |
| Flexor digitorum profundus | | | | |
| and sublimis* | | X | X | |
| First dorsal interosseus* | | X | | |
| Extensor pollicis longus | | | | |
| and brevis* | | | | X |
| Abductor pollicis brevis* | | | X | |
| Adductor pollicis* | | X | | |
| Opponens pollicis* | | | X | |

Note: For muscles innervated by more than one root, the predominant root level is indicated by ++ and less important levels by +.
* Impaired motor functions in case 21.

|                   |          | Roots |     |     |     |     |
| Musculocutaneous  | Axillary | C5    | C6  | C7  | C8  | T1  |
| ---               | ---      | ---   | --- | --- | --- | --- |
|                   |          | + +   | +   |     |     |     |
|                   | X        |       | + + | +   |     |     |
| X                 |          | + +   | + + |     |     |     |
|                   |          | +     | + + |     |     |     |
|                   |          |       | +   | + + | +   |     |
|                   |          |       | + + | + + |     |     |
|                   |          |       |     | +   | + + | +   |
|                   |          | +     | + + |     |     |     |
|                   |          |       |     | + + | +   |     |
|                   |          |       | + + | + + |     |     |
|                   |          |       | + + | + + |     |     |
|                   |          |       |     | + + | +   |     |
|                   |          |       |     | +   | + + | +   |
|                   |          |       |     |     | +   | + + |
|                   |          |       |     | + + | +   |     |
|                   |          |       |     |     | +   | + + |
|                   |          |       |     |     | +   | + + |
|                   |          |       |     |     | +   | + + |

Anisocoria is never due to an afferent pupillary defect. Fibers from the retinal ganglion cells, which convey light brightness information, bypass the lateral geniculate nucleus to synapse in the pretectal nucleus. Fibers then pass to both Edinger-Westphal nuclei. Parasympathetic fibers from this midbrain nucleus travel in the substance of the oculomotor nerve to innervate the iris sphincter muscle (Fig. 21-4A). Bilateral and equal Edinger-Westphal innervation ensures bilateral symmetric pupillary constriction to a unilateral light stimulus. Pupil diameters thus remain equal for retinal, optic nerve, or optic tract lesions. Damage to the optic radiation or occipital (visual) cortex does not alter the pupillary light reflex.

Efferent pupillary defects follow injury to parasympathetic or sympathetic pathways. Parasympathetic stimulation causes pupil constriction, whereas sympathetic stimulation causes dilatation. Damage to these autonomic fibers produces effects on pupil size that are opposite to those of stimulation. Sympathetic neurons descend from the hypothalamus to lower cervical and upper thoracic regions of the spinal cord. After synapsing in the intermediolateral columns, sympathetic fibers exit at the T1 level to enter the paravertebral sympathetic chain and course near the apex of the lung. After a second synapse in the superior cervical ganglion at the base of the skull, fibers to the eye are applied to the internal carotid artery. Sympathetic nerves to sweat glands of the upper face also follow the internal carotid artery. Intracranially, fibers to the pupil travel with branches of the ophthalmic division of the trigeminal nerve. Other fibers innervate the smooth muscle (Müller's muscle) of the eyelids. Sympathetic damage causes Horner's triad of pupillomiosis, eyelid ptosis, and facial anhidrosis (absence of sweating). The ocular sympathetic pathways are shown in Figure 21-4B. Note that sympathetic fibers are vulnerable at a number of intracranial and extracranial sites. For example, lateral medullary infarction involving descending sympathetic neurons (see case 5) is one cause of Horner's syndrome.

Next, decide whether parasympathetic (usually oculomotor nerve) or sympathetic damage caused the patient's anisocoria. This determination depends on which is abnormal: the smaller right pupil or the larger left pupil. Examination of the pupils in both bright and dim light often provides the answer. In bright light, the right pupil was 1.5 mm; the left, 2 mm. Five seconds after lights were dimmed, the left and right pupillary diameters were 3 and 7 mm, respectively. Twenty seconds later, the diameters were 5 and 7 mm.

Is the defect parasympathetic or sympathetic? What is the anatomic diagnosis?

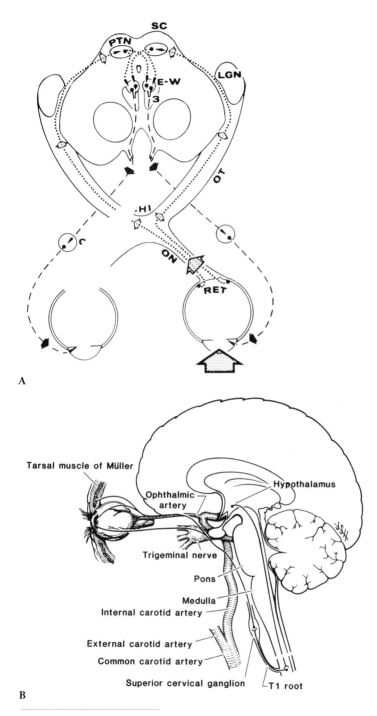

FIGURE 21-4.
See Fig. 6-2 (p. 73) for key to abbreviations. Part A reproduced with permission from Glaser, J. *Neuro-ophthalmology*. Hagerstown, Md.: Harper & Row, 1978.

In this patient anisocoria was accentuated in dim light, more so immediately after lights had been dimmed. This finding is characteristic of Horner's syndrome, and the smaller right pupil was therefore abnormal. For a parasympathetic defect, anisocoria would have been diminished in the dark. Right ptosis is another sympathetic defect; ipsilateral facial anhidrosis, suggested by the smooth, dry right forehead, completes the Horner's triad.

The anatomic diagnosis must be a lesion of the right C8–T1 nerve roots, severing upper extremity motor and sensory fibers and ocular sympathetic fibers. As sympathetic fibers do not enter the brachial plexus, damage to the lower trunk of the right plexus could not cause the concomitant Horner's syndrome.

The anatomic diagnosis for the patient's weakness and sensory loss could be confirmed by appropriate electrical studies. Electromyography either of the right arm or of the right upper extremity would show typical electrical features of denervation confined to muscles supplied by C8 and T1 roots.

However, these studies do not differentiate a C8–T1 root lesion from one of the lower trunk of the brachial plexus. Figure 21-5 shows how posterior (sensory) and anterior (motor) roots unite to form the mixed (sensory and motor) spinal nerve. The spinal nerve itself immediately divides into a smaller posterior ramus, conveying sensory and motor fibers to the back, and a larger anterior ramus which, for the upper extremities, joins other mixed roots in the brachial plexus. Figure 21-5 also shows the relation of the sympathetic ganglia and chain to the roots.

How might sensory nerve conduction studies or additional electromyographic studies help distinguish a C8–T1 lesion from one of the lower trunk of the brachial plexus?

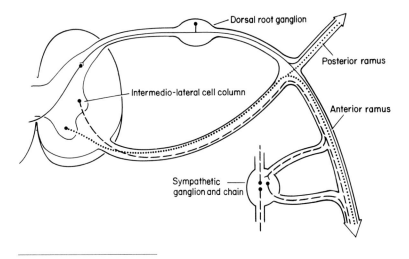

FIGURE 21-5.
Solid line: sensory nerve; dotted line: motor nerve; dashed line: sympathetic nerve.

If electromyography were to show denervation of the paraspinal muscles innervated by posterior rami of mixed spinal nerve roots, then the lesion would have to be proximal to the plexus. Similarly, if the anterior and posterior roots had been avulsed from the spinal cord, sensory nerve conduction velocities would remain normal despite complete anesthesia in the appropriate root distribution. Unlike the lower motor neuron whose cell body lies within the cord itself, sensory nerve fibers arise from dorsal root ganglia extrinsic to the cord (Fig. 21-5). Thus, sensory fibers, which remain in continuity with their cell bodies of origin, do not degenerate after root avulsion and are capable of normal impulse conduction.

Pharmacologic testing could confirm that the Horner's syndrome is due to a lesion located before the superior cervical ganglion. Damage to sympathetic fibers distal to the ganglion (i.e., postganglionic fibers) precludes input to adrenergic pupillary receptors, leading to a phenomenon known as denervation supersensitivity. Thus, adrenergic pharmacologic agents placed in the denervated eye will lead to pupillary dilatation at doses that do not significantly affect the normal eye. In addition, hydroxyamphetamine, a drug that acts to stimulate the release of norepinephrine from the postganglionic terminal in the iris, or cocaine, which blocks norepinephrine reuptake, normally causes pupillary dilatation. In this case, hydroxyamphetamine instilled by eyedrops caused pupillodilatation in the eye with the smaller pupil. Dilatation occurred because the lesion is in the second-order neuron (C8–T1 region of spinal cord to superior cervical ganglion), thus sparing the third-order neuron (superior cervical ganglion to the iris). Cocaine instillation to the eye caused no response because the input to the third-order neuron was diminished by the second-order neuron lesion.

What are the pathologic and neurologic differential diagnoses? What is the neurologic diagnosis?

Although many pathologic processes might involve nerve roots (e.g., herniated intervertebral discs, tumors), the history of a motorcycle accident strongly implies that the neurologic differential diagnosis should favor pathologic possibilities related to trauma. In this case, a traumatic avulsion at the time of the motorcycle accident of the C8–T1 nerve roots on the right side would be the most probable diagnosis. Damage to C8–T1 roots or to the lower trunk of the brachial plexus causes a pattern of upper extremity weakness commonly termed a Dejerine-Klumpke palsy. Injury to C5–C6 roots or to the upper trunk causes an Erb-Duchenne palsy. A Dejerine-Klumpke palsy or the more common Erb-Duchenne palsy may follow excessive traction on the brachial plexus, especially with hyperabduction of the arm or distraction of the head and shoulder, respectively. Motorcycle accidents are a common cause of brachial plexus injuries in adults. Infants are especially susceptible to these injuries during a difficult birth.

**Case 22**

**Double Vision and Facial Numbness**

## Case 22

Two weeks before hospitalization a 23-year-old man developed frontal head pain. There also was drooping of the left eyelid. When he held his eyelid open, he noted double vision when attempting to look in any direction other than straight ahead. The next week he noted numbness of his right forehead when combing his hair. Both ptosis and diplopia worsened progressively.

The patient was alert and oriented, with fluent and well-articulated speech. Muscle tone, strength, and coordination, tendon reflexes, trunk and limb sensation, and gait were normal. Babinski's signs were absent. Visual fields were intact. The right pupil was 3 mm in diameter and noramlly reactive to light. The left pupil was 5 mm in diameter and did not react to light. Marked left eyelid ptosis was present. When the eyelid was lifted, it was apparent that the patient could not move his left eye from its straight-ahead position. Movements of the right eye were normal. There was decreased pinprick sensation in the distribution areas of the ophthalmic (first) and maxillary (second) divisions of the left trigeminal nerve (Fig. 22-1).

What is the anatomic diagnosis?

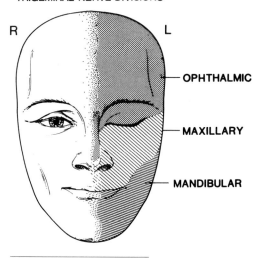

FIGURE 22-1.

The left oculomotor, trochlear, and abducens nerves must be involved to cause total paralysis of the patient's left eye. An intrinsic brainstem lesion, affecting the ophthalmic and maxillary divisions of the trigeminal nerve and these oculomotor nerves, would extend from the midbrain to the lower pons. However, such an extensive lesion should also affect other structures. Might a lesion outside the brainstem affect the pathway of these four cranial nerves?

Figure 22-2, a lateral brainstem view with the cerebellum removed, illustrates some of the cranial nerves as they exit from the brainstem. The oculomotor nerve exits from the midbrain and courses anteriorly, lateral to the posterior clinoid processes in the lateral wall of the cavernous sinus, and then passes through the superior orbital fissure to the eye. The trochlear nerve exits at the dorsal aspect of the midbrain. It then courses ventrally and anteriorly under the tentorium to join the oculomotor nerve in the lateral wall of the cavernous sinus, and then passes through the superior orbital fissure to the orbit. The abducens nerve leaves the ventral aspect of the brainstem at the pontomedullary junction and courses superiorly and anteriorly to join the oculomotor and trochlear nerves in the lateral wall of the cavernous sinus.

The ophthalmic division of the trigeminal nerve leaves the gasserian ganglion to join the oculomotor, trochlear, and abducens nerves in the lateral wall of the cavernous sinus; it also passes through the superior orbital fissure to the orbit. The maxillary division branches off the gasserian ganglion and courses inferiorly and then anteriorly. It enters the posterior portion of the cavernous sinus before exiting from the skull through the foramen rotundum. The mandibular division descends after leaving the gasserian ganglion to exit through the foramen ovale without passing through the cavernous sinus.

What is the anatomic diagnosis?

The only anatomic site shared by the oculomotor, trochlear, abducens nerves and the ophthalmic and maxillary divisions of the trigeminal nerve is the cavernous sinus (all these structures pass through the superior orbital fissure except the maxillary division of the trigeminal nerve). This is shown in Figure 22-2.

**W**hat is the pathologic differential diagnosis?

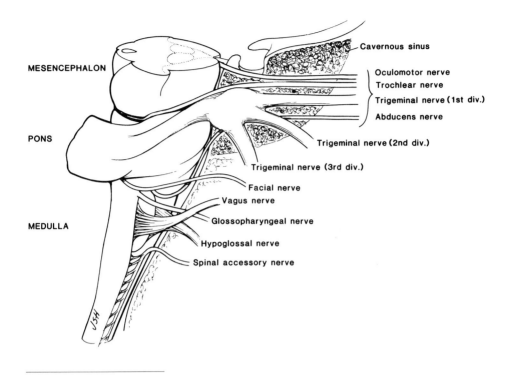

FIGURE 22-2.

The cavernous sinus (Fig. 22-3) contains a venous plexus, which may be a focus for infection, thrombophlebitis, and thrombosis. Abnormal communications may occur between the arterial and venous systems in the cavernous sinus, i.e., carotid cavernous sinus fistula. Since this venous plexus is in communication with ophthalmic veins, signs of venous congestion (e.g., proptosis, chemosis, and cyanosis and edema of the forehead and eyelid) usually occur with venous involvement. A portion of the internal carotid artery also lies within the cavernous sinus. Aneurysms in this region may cause the clinical findings just discussed. Tumors arising from the meninges forming the wall of the cavernous sinus (meningiomas) may cause this clinical syndrome, as may metastatic tumors or tumors invading from adjacent structures.

What is the neurologic differential diagnosis? Since there are no signs of venous congestion, carotid cavernous fistula and cavernous sinus thrombosis are unlikely. The acute onset of pain and ophthalmoplegia makes aneurysm more likely than tumor. A CT scan showed a circumscribed contrast-enhancing mass present in the left cavernous sinus. A cerebral angiogram confirmed this to be an aneurysm of carotid artery within the cavernous sinus.

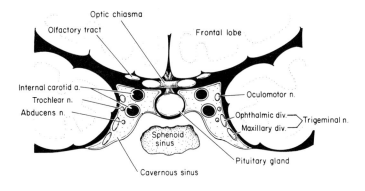

FIGURE 22-3.

**Case 23**

# Facial Weakness

## Case 23

A 44-year-old woman awoke to discover an aching sensation of her right mastoid and ear. When she looked in the mirror, she was alarmed to see that her face was asymmetric. The right side of her face drooped, and when she tried to smile the right side of her mouth did not move (Fig. 23-1). Her right palpebral fissure was wider than the left, and she was tearing from her right eye. As she ate her breakfast, she found that food became caught in her right cheek, and fluids dribbled out of the right side of her mouth.

Her vital signs were normal, and she was alert and oriented. Her speech was slurred when she tried to repeat such sounds as "me-me-me." The right nasolabial fold was markedly flattened, and there were no creases or wrinkles on the right side of the face. The right palpebral fissure width was 10 mm and the left was 7 mm (normal), and she continued to have tearing from her right eye. On forced eye closure, both eyes deviated up and out (the normal Bell's phenomenon). Even on vigorous attempts to close her eyes, 3 mm of sclera still showed on the right. When asked to look up, she wrinkled the left forehead well, but there were no wrinkles of the right forehead. She could not drink through a straw or whistle. Snapping fingers by her right ear caused no discomfort, and she was able to hear the ticking of a watch in each ear. She was unable to perceive sweet and salty solutions dabbed on the right side of her tongue but readily identified these when they were applied to the left side. Other cranial nerve functions, sensation, strength, coordination, tendon reflexes, and gait were normal.

Where would a lesion be to produce these findings?

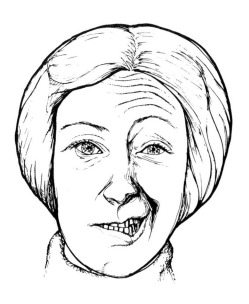

FIGURE 23-1.

Facial muscles other than the muscles of mastication are innervated by the facial nucleus and nerve. The facial nucleus lies in the dorsal-lateral region of the lower pons. Supranuclear input from the cerebral cortex is predominantly bilateral for muscles of the forehead and unilateral for the lower face. These supranuclear fibers cross just above the level of the facial nucleus (solid line, Fig. 23-2A). Motoneurons from the facial nucleus pass through the paramedian pontine reticular formation and, as the internal genu of the seventh nerve, loop around the nucleus of the abducens nerve, forming the facial colliculus in the floor of the fourth ventricle (dashed line, Fig. 23-2A). After making this loop, these motoneurons are joined by neurons from the nucleus solitarius, which subserve taste on the anterior two-thirds of the tongue, and by neurons from the superior salivatory nucleus, which convey parasympathetic input to the salivary and lacrimal glands. The nerve fascicle then passes between the facial nucleus and the descending nucleus and tract of the trigeminal nerve, where general somatic afferent fibers of the trigeminal nerve merge with the facial nerve fascicle. These fibers convey cutaneous sensory impulses from the region of the mastoid and the external auditory canal. Fibers for somatesthetic sensation, taste on the anterior two-thirds of the tongue, and salivary and lacrimal gland functions form the portion of the facial nerve called the intermediate nerve. The intermediate nerve emerges between the vestibular portion of the vestibulocochlear cranial nerve and the facial motor root at the cerebellopontine angle.

The facial nerve then passes with the auditory nerve through the internal acoustic canal and separates from the vestibulocochlear nerve to enter the facial canal in the petrous portion of the temporal bone. It then makes an abrupt posterior bend (the external genu) and runs in the medial wall of the tympanic cavity just above the oval window. The geniculate ganglion lies in the region of the external genu, where the greater superficial petrosal nerve leaves. This branch eventually innervates the lacrimal gland (Fig. 23-2B). After further descent in the petrous portion of the temporal bone, a branch is given off to the stapedius muscle. In response to loud noise, the stapedius dampens the stapes in the middle ear thereby preventing damage to the cochlea. For lesions of the facial nerve proximal to the stapedius innervation, moderately loud noises are quite disagreeable (hyperacusis). Distal to the branch to the stapedius muscle is the chorda tympani, which innervates the submaxillary gland and carries taste information from the anterior two-thirds of the tongue. Before the nerve exits through the stylomastoid foramen to innervate the muscles of facial expression, a cutaneous branch is given off to the external ear.

**W**hat is the anatomic diagnosis for the patient's symptoms and signs?

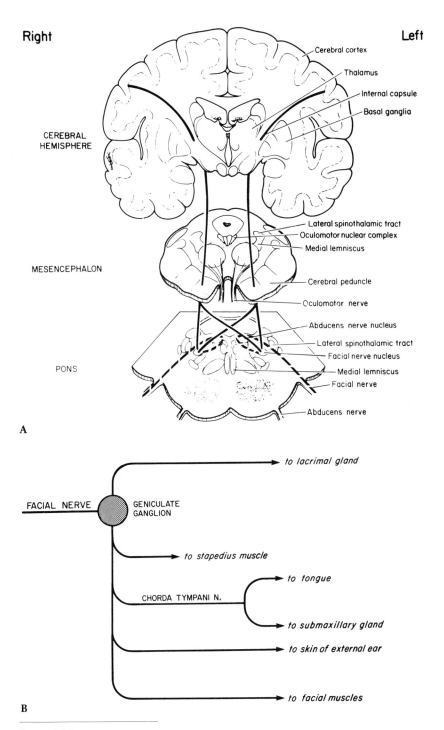

FIGURE 23-2.

The absence of cerebellar, corticospinal, and spinothalamic signs implies that the lesion is not within the brainstem. Thus, the lesion must affect the peripheral portion of the facial nerve. Since the muscles of facial expression are paralyzed on the right, taste is lost on the anterior two-thirds of the tongue, and there is pain the region of the mastoid, the lesion must be proximal to the chorda tympani. Tearing was evident, indicating the presence of facial nerve function from the brainstem up to the greater superficial petrosal nerve, and there was no hyperacusis, implying that input to the stapedius muscle is intact. Thus, the lesion must be distal to the branch to the stapedius muscle.

The pathologic differential diagnosis would include idiopathic inflammatory disorders of the facial nerve (i.e., Bell's palsy), primary or metastatic tumor, abscess, granulomatous disease (sarcoidosis), or basilar skull fracture. Since there were no findings in the history or physical examination to suggest tumor, trauma, or infection, a presumptive diagnosis of Bell's palsy is the most likely possibility for the neurologic diagnosis.

Bell's palsy is a common disorder of the facial nerve of unknown cause (possibly viral). The onset is abrupt, and progression occurs over days. For incomplete lesions there will be gradual recovery within 3 to 6 weeks. During recovery, the nerves may regenerate aberrantly such that the salivary or lacrimal glands are innervated by the motor portion of the nerve, causing inappropriate tearing and salivation when the muscles innervated by the facial nerve are used (crocodile tears). Aberrant regeneration within the motor system of the nerve may cause such a phenomenon as eye closure when the patient attempts to use muscles of the lower face, as in smiling.

Over the course of the following six weeks, the patient made a full recovery, thus substantiating the neurologic diagnosis of Bell's palsy.

**Case 24**

**Difficulty Walking and Urinary Bladder Dysfunction**

## Case 24

Over the past 4 months a 45-year-old man had experienced increasing difficulty walking. At first he would stumble over his right foot, particularly when stepping up onto a curb. Three months previously he had noticed a "deep aching" pain vaguely localized to the perineum, at first intermittent but later present almost constantly. More recently, his legs had felt weak, and he described a "numb" feeling in his buttocks. He denied increased frequency of urination, but on several occasions he was surprised to find that his underwear was wet. A month previously an antibiotic had been prescribed for a urinary tract infection. He also admitted that he had become impotent.

His vital signs were normal. He was anxious but alert and oriented. Speech and language were intact. General physical findings were significant for an enlarged bladder. He denied a need to urinate. There was no tenderness to percussion of the spine. Cranial nerve functions, coordination (finger-nose-finger and heel-knee-shin tasks), and upper extremity tone, strength, sensation, and tendon reflexes were normal.

As he walked, there was exaggerated flexion of the right hip, during which the right foot remained plantar flexed. In descent, he quickly flung his right lower leg forward, thereby passively dorsiflexing the dangling right foot, which then audibly slapped the floor. He was unable to stand on his toes on the right side or on his heel on the left. Inspection of his shoes showed that the toe of the right sole was more worn than that of the left.

The sharp anterior border of the right tibia was visibly prominent from the loss of tibialis anterior muscle bulk. The right thigh circumference was 2 cm less than the left (wasting of the right quadriceps muscle), and the left calf was 1 cm less than the right (wasting of the left gastrocnemius and soleus muscles). There was asymmetric weakness of each leg (Table 24-1).

Lower extremity sensation was impaired bilaterally to all modalities (pinprick, light touch with a wisp of cotton, vibrating tuning fork) over the left posterior thigh and asymmetrically over both buttocks (Fig. 24-1). Right quadriceps and left gastrocnemius tendon reflexes were diminished, and Babinski's signs were absent. Rectal tone was diminished on digital examination. There was no contraction of the external sphincter when the perianal region was pricked with a pin and, similarly, no bulbocavernous muscle contraction (palpated on the perineum and during digital rectal examination) when the glans of the penis was pricked (i.e., no anal wink and no bulbocavernous reflex). Abdominal and cremasteric reflexes were normal.

Begin by considering the patient's gait. What functional anatomic system is impaired?

Table 24-1.
Patient's lower extremity strength

| Muscle | Strength* Left | Right |
|---|---|---|
| Femoral nerve | | |
| Iliopsoas | 5 | 5 |
| Quadriceps | 5 | 4 |
| Obturator nerve | | |
| Adductors longus and magnus | 5 | 5 |
| Superior gluteal nerve | | |
| Gluteus medius and minimus, and tensor fasciae latae | 5 | 4 |
| Inferior gluteal nerve | | |
| Gluteus maximus | 5 | 5 |
| Sciatic and tibial nerves | | |
| Hamstring | 5 | 5 |
| Gastrocnemius/soleus | 4 | 5 |
| Tibialis posterior | 5 | 4 |
| Flexor digitorum longus | 4 | 5 |
| Flexor hallucis longus | 4 | 5 |
| Small muscles of foot | 4 | 5 |
| Peroneal branch of sciatic nerve | | |
| Tibialis anterior | 5 | 2 |
| Extensor digitorum longus | 5 | 5 |
| Extensor hallucis longus | 5 | 5 |
| Extensor digitorum brevis | 5 | 5 |
| Peroneus longus and brevis | 5 | 5 |

* Grades of muscle strength: 0 = no contraction; 1 = contraction of muscle but no movement of joint; 2 = movement of joint but not against gravity; 3 = movement against gravity but without any additional resistance; 4 = movement against added resistance but still weak; and 5 = normal strength.

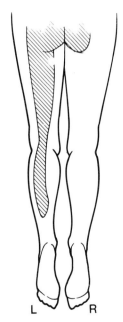

FIGURE 24-1.

## Case 24

Disorders of gait are usually caused by disturbances in motor or sensory systems. Nonneurogenic gait disorders caused, for example, by pain or orthopedic abnormalities are usually obvious. One must be aware, however, that the underlying cause of some orthopedic problems, such as scoliosis or a club foot, may actually be neurologic.

The particular functional system implicated in a disordered gait is readily identified on the basis of associated neurologic findings, such as muscle tone and strength, tendon reflexes, coordination, and sensation. In most cases, however, observation of the gait itself suggests an anatomic diagnosis. Several examples follow.

Proximal weakness is a feature of most muscle diseases (myopathies), and hip weakness will cause a characteristic waddling gait. The weakened thigh abductors are unable to stabilize the pelvis as the leg is lifted from the ground, permitting a drop of the contralateral side of the pelvis. The waddle is, thus, due to pelvic rocking with each step. To compensate for weakened paraspinal muscles, the posture becomes increasingly lordotic (swayback). This posture represents a compensatory backward shift in the center of gravity such that the trunk comes to lie directly over the hips. The myopathic patient may also be unable to rise from the floor or from a low chair or, in attempting to stand, may place the hand on the thigh to support the trunk (Gowers' sign).

Extrapyramidal disorders (for example, Parkinson's disease) cause characteristic abnormalities of gait. Parkinsonian features are apparent even before the patient attempts to walk: kyphotic (stooped) posture, a blank facial expression with infrequent blinking, "pill-rolling" tremor (four or five movements per second) of the resting fingers and thumb, and a paucity and slowness of other spontaneous movements (bradykinesia). Indeed, severe bradykinesia may prevent the patient from being able to initiate the first step. The patient may even step or fall backward (retropulsion). The gait is narrow-based (i.e., feet are close together), and steps are short and shuffling. The extent of the accompanying arm swing is limited. Steps may begin slowly but rapidly increase in tempo (festination).

For the spastic gait of a unilateral corticospinal system lesion, the stiffly extended affected leg must be circumducted in an arc to compensate for incomplete hip and knee flexion. In contrast, the upper extremity is maintained in a position of flexion. Disease of the midline cerebellum preferentially impairs lower extremity and truncal coordination, causing a wide-based, reeling ataxic gait. Tandem gait (heel-to-toe walking) is then impossible.

The present patient's gait differs from those described. A slapping gait is seen with marked weakness of ankle dorsiflexion. Patients unable to dorsiflex the foot are in danger of falling, as slight elevations become obstacles to catch the dangling toe. To raise the entire foot, they must increase the degree of hip and knee flexion; hence, the high-stepping gait. In addition, they tend to fling the leg forward, throwing the foot upward so that it lands flat on the ground with a slapping sound. A stomping gait occurs with proprioceptive loss (certain polyneuropathies, and diseases, such as tabes dorsalis, that affect the posterior columns of the spinal cord). The gait is caused by the patient's attempt to compensate for not knowing the exact position of the foot and leg. The foot drops heavily on the ground to augment proprioceptive input. Unlike the "slapping" gait of distal weakness, however, the foot does not dangle limply from the overly flexed leg.

For this patient the neurologic examination confirmed wasting and marked weakness of his right tibialis anterior muscle, causing his foot drop and steppage gait. There was also selective weakness of other lower extremity muscles (see Table 24-1). This pattern of selective muscle involvement does not occur with disease of the upper motoneuron, lower motoneuron, neuromuscular junction, or muscle.

Consider his motor, sensory, and reflex findings. Table 24-2 lists some lower extremity muscles and their patterns of innervation. Is the anatomic diagnosis that of root, plexus, or peripheral nerve?

Table 24-2.
Segmental Innervation of Lower Extremity Muscles

| Muscle | Segment* |
|---|---|
| *Femoral nerve* | |
|   Iliopsoas | L1, L2, (L3) |
|   Quadriceps | (L2), L3, L4 |
| *Obturator nerve* | |
|   Adductors longus and magnus | L2, L3, (L4) |
| *Superior gluteal nerve* | |
|   Gluteus medius and minimus | L4, L5, (S1) |
|   Tensor fasciae latae | L4, L5, (S1) |
| *Inferior gluteal nerve* | |
|   Gluteus maximus | L5, S1, (S2) |
| *Sciatic and tibial nerves* | |
|   Hamstring | (L5), S1, (S2) |
|   Gastrocnemius/soleus | S1, S2 |
|   Tibialis posterior | L4, L5 |
|   Flexor digitorum longus | (L5), S1, S2 |
|   Flexor hallucis longus | (L5), S1, S2 |
|   Small muscles of foot | S1, S2 |
| *Peroneal branch of sciatic nerve* | |
|   Tibialis anterior | L4 (L5) |
|   Extensor digitorum longus | L5, (S1) |
|   Extensor hallucis longus | L5, (S1) |
|   Extensor digitorum brevis | L5, S1 |
|   Peroneus longus and brevis | L5, S1 |

* Parenthetical listing for minor source of innervation.

The deficits are not those of a peripheral nerve lesion. For example, the right tibialis anterior muscle is quite weak, but the right extensor hallucis longus (the dorsiflexor of the big toe), which is innervated by the same branch of the sciatic nerve as is the tibialis anterior, remains strong. Unilateral abnormalities characterize plexus lesions, but this patient has bilateral signs. On the other hand, involvement of the right L4 motor root and bilateral sacral motor and sensory roots (S3–5 on the right; S2–5 on the left) might explain his disorder.

Is this anatomic diagnosis of bilateral noncontiguous root involvement more parsimonious than bilateral lumbosacral plexus lesions? The affirmative answer is explained by the anatomy of the lower spine, cord, and roots. Developmentally, the vertebral column elongates faster than the cord that it envelops. At the time of birth, the lower end of the cord is usually at the level of the L3 vertebral body; for adults this level is at L1 or L2 (Fig. 24-2). (For this reason, a properly performed lumbar puncture, in which the needle penetrates the dura between the L4 and L5 vertebral bodies, ordinarily poses no hazard to the cord itself.) Regardless of developmental stage, a given spinal root exists at the same intervertebral level. The adult spinal canal thus contains the elongated lumbar, sacral, and coccygeal roots, which descend from the lower cord to their respective levels of exit through bony foramina. In aggregate, these roots resemble a horse's tail, and the term *cauda equina* is derived from this description. Intradural lesions of the lower spinal canal often affect the cauda equina. Pain, a common symptom, may be referred to the back, thighs, perineum, rectum, or genitalia, regions innervated by nerves derived from the cauda equina. Symptoms and signs are often asymmetric, depending on the particular combination of involved roots. At times the initial abnormalities are unilateral, making especially difficult the differentiation between a plexus or peripheral nerve lesion.

Are the patient's bladder and sexual disturbances consistent with the provisional anatomic diagnosis of a cauda equina lesion, or do they implicate dysfunction at a higher level of the nervous system? Begin with his bladder disturbance. What are the expected symptoms and signs of bladder dysfunction of peripheral (root, plexus, nerve) and central (cord, brain) lesions?

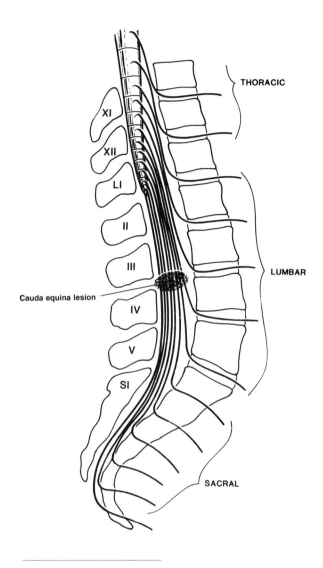

FIGURE 24-2.

The complex act of micturition, under reflex and voluntary control, requires relaxation of perineal muscles, tensing of abdominal muscles to increase intraabdominal pressure, contraction of the interlacing detrusor muscle fibers of the bladder, and relaxation of the urethral sphincters. Unilateral neurologic damage is usually asymptomatic, but bilateral lesions at several nervous system levels can affect bladder function by altering detrusor or sphincter function.

Diffuse cerebral abnormalities (for example, the confusional state of metabolic encephalopathies) and focal injury to the cerebral hemispheres (particularly bilateral lesions of the medial aspect of the frontal lobe) interface with the voluntary initiation and control of micturition. Corticospinal fibers and fibers from the brainstem reticular formation are important for sphincter and detrusor functioning. Intracranial or spinal interruption of upper motoneuron fibers for the detrusor muscle may cause a spastic bladder. Reflex detrusor contractions then begin at relatively small bladder volumes, giving rise to urgency, frequency, and incontinence. Lower motoneuron and sensory fibers important for micturition exit and enter the sacral cord. Lower motoneuron lesions (parasympathetic detrusor neurons arise from the intermediolateral gray columns) and peripheral nerve lesions often cause a hypotonic bladder. The force of the urine stream is decreased, and the distended bladder fails to empty completely. Residual urine proves to be a fertile bacterial medium, and infections of the urinary system are common. Sensory lesions (either peripheral nerve or in the spinal cord) affect normal reflexive detrusor contractions. The sensation of bladder fullness will be lost, causing overflow incontinence of small quantities of urine. Because CNS pathways modulating detrusor function are separate from those for the urethral sphincter, a spastic bladder need not always imply a spastic sphincter, and vice versa.

Studies of detrusor and sphincter functions are augmented by cystometry and urethral electromyography, respectively. The former technique involves continuous monitoring of intravesicular pressure as a fluid or a gas is instilled into the bladder.

For this patient bladder dysfunction proved to be that of a hypotonic deafferented bladder. The history suggested overflow incontinence, with incomplete bladder emptying predisposing to his urinary tract infection. Furthermore, although the patient denied a sensation of fullness, the bladder was palpably enlarged on examination. Additional studies were done. As the bladder was filled for cystometry, there were no detrusor contractions, and the patient reported no sensation of fullness.

Sacral roots are also important for defecation and for sexual functions. The history of impotence and findings of decreased anal sphincter tone on digital examination, absent anal wink, and absent bulbocavernous reflex support an anatomic diagnosis that includes bilateral sacral root involvment. Thus, the lesion involves multiple roots bilaterally, the cauda equina syndrome.

The pathologic differential diagnosis includes pathologic alterations of tissue normally present in the region of the cauda equina. Meningiomas can arise from the meningeal coverings of the spinal cord, neurofibromas and schwannomas from the nerve roots, and ependymomas from ependymal cells of the filum terminale. A protruding intervertebral disc, a hematoma from ruptured blood vessels in the epidural space, and epidural or vertebral body abscesses or metastatic tumors can all compress the cauda equina. The 4-month history of progressive worsening favors an expanding mass lesion in the neurologic differential diagnosis. A hematoma or ruptured intervertebral disc is thus unlikely.

Myelography and magnetic resonance imaging scan of the spine revealed an intradural mass. The neurologic diagnosis, confirmed by histologic examination of the surgically resected tumor, was an ependymoma, a tumor derived from ependymal cells that line the central canal of the cord and the filum terminale.

# Index

# Index

Abducens nerve
  in abduction of left eye, 44
  in brainstem anatomy, 246
  dysconjugate gaze and, 178
  functions of, 94
  horizontal gaze and, 190
  left gaze paresis and, 32
  and paramedian pontine reticular formation activation, 208
  paresis of, increased intracranial pressure and, 194
Abductor digiti minimi, weakness of, 220, 222–223
Abductor pollicis, weakness of, 220, 222–223
Abscess, and increased intracranial pressure, 156
Acquired language disorders. See Aphasia
Adenoma, pituitary, prolactin secretion from, 96
Afferent pupillary defect, 72
  versus efferent, in anisocoria, 232, 235, 236
Afferent visual system
  anatomy of, 104
  pathway subserving, 74
Agraphesthesia, 80
Alexia
  versus illiteracy, 132
  lesion for, 130
  and right visual field loss, 126–133
Alpha motoneuron, reflexes and, 14
Amaurosis fugax, 136, 146
  pathologic differential diagnosis for, 148
Amygdaloid nuclei, in olfactory system anatomy, 102
Anesthesia, of the face, 62
Aneurysm
  of carotid artery, in cavernous sinus, 248
  ruptured, unconsciousness and, 194
Anhidrosis, facial
  in Horner's syndrome, 67
  sympathetic damage and, 236
Anisocoria
  afferent versus efferent pupillary defects in, 232, 235, 236
  dilatation lag in, 238
  traumatic weakness and numbness with, 228–241
Ankle dorsiflexion, gait disorders and, 263
Anomia, 108
  perisylvian language core and, 142
Anosmia, factitious, 200
Anterior cerebral artery
  anatomic localization of occlusion in, 166
  cingulate herniation and, 210
  infarction of, 54
  strokes and, 88
Anterior circulation
  in brain arterial system, 88
  disease signs and symptoms in, 89
Anterior communicating arteries, and optic chiasm compression, 96
Anterior horn cell
  denervation, in traumatic weakness, 230
  lesion of, 218
Anterior ramus, spinal nerve and, 238
Anterior spinal artery, anatomic localization of occlusion in, 166
Aphasia, 108
  anomic, 108
    perisylvian language core and, 142
  and auditory comprehension, 112
  and Broca's area. See Broca's area
  conduction, 112, 113, 133
  and cortical involvement, 109
  and fluency of speech, 110
  mixed transcortical, 133
  sensory modalities and, 109
  stroke and, 114
  types of, 112, 113
  and Wernicke's area. See Wernicke's area
Apneustic breathing, 194
  coma and, 210
Apraxia
  cortical disconnection syndromes and, 146
  sympathetic, 133
  lesion location for, 146
Arcuate fasciculus
  language system and, 109, 110
  and motor response mediation, 146
Arteriovenous malformations, hemisphere involvement in, 194
Artery
  anterior cerebral. See Anterior cerebral artery
  anterior communicating, and optic chiasm compression, 96
  anterior spinal, occlusion in, 166
  basilar. See Basilar artery
  common carotid, atherosclerotic changes in, 148
  distribution in brain, 88
  internal carotid. See Internal carotid artery
  ophthalmic, occlusion in
    left visual field loss and, 88
    platelet-thrombin embolus in, 148
  small end, occlusion of, 166
  superior cerebral, occlusion in, 166
  and supply regions in the brain, 166
  vertebral. See Vertebral artery
Astereognosis, 80

Astrocytoma, 44
  spinal cord lesion and, 20
Asymmetry, facial, 252
Ataxia, 60, 67
  factitious, and Romberg's sign, 201
  of gait and trunk, 152–157
  and ipsilateral cerebellum lesions, 66
  and lateral zone of the cerebellum lesion, 162
Ataxic breathing, 194
Atherosclerosis
  amaurosis fugax and, 148
  and predilection for lesion sites, 88
Atrophy, cerebral, subdural hematoma and, 56
Attention, deficits in, 118, 122
Auditory comprehension
  apraxia and, 144
  as parameter in aphasia, 110, 112
Auditory cortex, and "cortically deaf" patients, 110
Auditory nerve, facial nerve pathway and, 254
Aurae, in seizures, 100
Automatisms, stereotyped and reactive, 102
Avulsion, traumatic, of C8–T1 nerve roots, 240–241

Babinski's sign, 12, 14
Baroreception, 122
Basilar artery
  occlusion of, 166
    and left-sided weakness, 180
  in posterior circulation, 88
Basis pontis, lesion of, in left arm ataxia and weakness, 164
Behavior alteration, 100–104
Bell's palsy, 256
Bell's phenomenon
  and forced eye closure, 252
  in unconsciousness, 198
Biceps, innervation of, 14
Bitemporal hemianopsia
  afferent visual system and, 74, 75
  optic chiasm compression and, 96
Bladder
  dysfunction. See Urinary bladder dysfunction
  hypotonic deafferented, 268
  spastic, 268
Blinking, and abnormal corneal reflexes, 176
Blood, in skull, 156
Blood vessels
  distribution in brain, 88
  occlusion of. See Vascular occlusion
Brachial plexus
  Dejerine-Klumpke palsy and, 241

  nerve root lesion differentiation and, 238
  in neural anatomy, 220
  traumatic nerve damage to, 230, 232
Brachium conjunctivum, lesion of, in left arm ataxia and weakness, 164
Bradykinesia, gait disorders and, 262
Brain
  artery distribution to, 88
  lesions in, language difficulty and, 109
  skull anatomy and, 156
  tumor of, symptoms associated with, 86
Brainstem
  corticospinal fibers in, 52, 140
  facial nerve axons in, 26
  involvement in unresponsiveness, 206
  lateral view of, 246, 247
  lesions of
    "crossed paralysis" and, 30
    differential diagnosis of, 67
Brainstem reticular activating system, in consciousness, 172
Breathing. See also Respiration, alteration in
  apneustic, 194
  coma and, 210
  ataxic, 194, 195
  lower pontine–upper medulla stage, 210
Bridging cortical veins
  shearing of, 56
  subdural hematoma and, 56
Brightness, and pupillary light reflex, 72
Broca's area
  anatomy of, 109
  function of, 110
  and left middle cerebral artery occlusion, 148
  lesion of, and sympathetic apraxia, 146
  nonfluent speech and, 144
  oral-facial apraxia and, 146
Brodmann's cortical areas, 82
Brown-Séquard syndrome, 18, 76
Bulbar musculature, speech difficulty and, 138
Bulbocavernous muscle reflex, walking difficulty and, 260

C8–T1 nerve roots
  and brachial plexus, lesion differentiation and, 238
  muscle weakness and, 232, 234–235
  traumatic avulsion of, 240–141
Calcarine cortex, afferent visual system and, 74, 75
Caloric testing, 192, 203
Carotid artery
  common, atherosclerotic changes in, 148

# Index

Carotid artery—*Continued*
  internal. *See* Internal carotid artery
Carotid cavernous sinus fistula, facial numbness and, 248
Carpal tunnel syndrome, 224
Cauda equina
  lesion, walking difficulty and, 266
  syndrome, 268
Cavernous sinus
  in brainstem anatomy, 246
  facial numbness and, 248
  oculomotor nerve and, 94
Central nervous system
  anatomy of, 13
    cerebellar cortex, 160
    corticospinal tract, 14, 15
    deep cerebellar nuclei, 160
    lateral spinothalamic tract, 16, 17
    medial lemniscus, 18, 19
  Cheyne-Stokes respirations and, 194
Central neurogenic hyperventilation, coma and, 210
Central transtentorial herniation, 210
Cerebellopontine angle, intermediate nerve and, 254
Cerebellum
  lateral zone of, 164
  longitudinal zones of, 154
Cerebral atrophy, subdural hematoma and, 56
Cerebral cortex
  and cortical sensations, 82
  corticospinal fibers in, 52, 140
  and supranuclear input to facial nucleus, 244
  and zones of cerebellum, 154
Cerebral hemispheres
  and brainstem reticular activating system, in consciousness, 172
  focal damage to, 123
  left, language difficulty and, 109
    differential diagnosis in, 114
  lesions in, facial weakness and, 28
  right, language difficulty and, 109
Cerebral peduncle, in voluntary gaze pathway, 208
Cerebral vascular disease, left arm weakness and, 166
Cerebrospinal fluid (CSF)
  obstructed flow, increased intracranial pressure and, 194
  in skull, 156
Cervical spinal cord lesion, right-sided weakness and, 14
Cheyne-Stokes respirations, 184
  in anatomic diagnosis of unconsciousness, 194
Chorda tympani, facial nerve pathway and, 254

Ciliary ganglion (CG), in pupillary light reflex pathway, 72
Cingulate herniation, 210
Circulation, anterior and posterior, 88
Claw hand deformity, 216
Clumsiness
  cerebellar dysfunction and, 66
  of gait, 152–156
  of left arm, 160–166
  of left hand, 136–148
  of right arm, 60, 67
Cocaine, and pupillary dilation, 240
Coma, central transtentorial herniation and, 210
Commands, verbal, 146
Common carotid artery, atherosclerotic changes in, 148
Common peroneal nerve, conduction vulnerability site for, 224
Comprehension. *See* Auditory comprehension
Compression, of spinal cord, 16
  Hodgkin's lymphoma and, 20
Conduction aphasia, 112, 133
Conduction block, in right-handed weakness and sensory loss, 224
Confrontational visual field testing, in double vision, 92
Conjugate gaze
  systems involved in, 178
  volitional, 32
Consciousness. *See also* Unconsciousness
  depression of, 170, 172
  systems required for, 172
Constriction, of pupils, 72
Conversion reaction, unconsciousness and, 200
Convexities, cerebral corticospinal fibers' origin in, 52
Corneal reflex
  abnormality in, and right facial weakness, 176
  and trigeminal nerve mediation, 62
Corona radiata, in left-sided weakness, 82
Corpus callosum
  and motor response mediation, 146
  visual input and, 130
Cortex
  auditory, and "cortically deaf" patients, 110
  calcarine, afferent visual system and, 74, 75
  cerebral. *See* Cerebral cortex
  motor
    apraxia and, 146
    lesion of, 146
    orbital frontal, 102

premotor, lesion of, 146
somatosensory, 82
Cortical disconnection syndromes, 132, 133. *See also* Alexia
apraxia and, 146
Corticobulbar fibers
lesion of, 28
and left facial weakness, 188
left-sided weakness and, 206
right-sided weakness and, 28
pathway to facial nucleus, 42
Corticobulbar pathway, and pain mediation, 188
Corticocerebellar fibers, lesion of, in left arm ataxia and weakness, 164
Corticospinal fibers
in brainstem, 52, 140
in cerebral cortex, 52, 140
origin of, 52
in spinal cord, 52
Corticospinal tract
ataxia and weakness of left arm and, 162
cerebral cortex and, 140
dysarthria and, 138
left facial weakness and, 26
and left-sided weakness, 174, 186, 206
lower extremity weakness and, 50
right, and left-sided weakness, 120
right-sided weakness and, 40, 41
route of, 14
Cranial nerves
in brainstem anatomy, 246
double vision and, 92
"Crossed analgesia," 60
"Crossed paralysis," 30
CSF. *See* Cerebrospinal fluid (CSF)
Cutaneous stimulus localization, 122

Decerebrate posturing, coma and, 210
Decerebrate response, 204, 206
Decussation, and corticospinal tract lesion
medullary, 50
pyramidal, 40
Dejerine-Klumpke palsy, 241
Demyelination
multiple sclerosis and, 76
ptosis and, 44
Dentate nucleus, and lateral zone of cerebellum, 164
Dermatomes, and sensory loss pattern, 232
Detrusor muscle, bladder dysfunction and, 268
Diencephalic dysfunction, central transtentorial herniation and, 210
Diplopia
and facial numbness, 244–248

galactorrhea and, 92–96
horizontal, 42
intracranial pressure and, 194
right-sided weakness and, 38–44
Discriminative sensations, and perceptual disturbances, 122
Disinhibition, Babinski's sign and, 14
Dizziness, 60–67
Doll's-head maneuver
dysconjugate gaze and, 170
pontine lesion in, 176
and left gaze paresis, 80, 84
ophthalmoplegia and, 204, 208
in unconsciousness, 198
Dorsal column. *See* Medial lemniscus
Dorsal interossei, weakness of, 220, 222–223
Dorsal root ganglion
in medial lemniscus system, 18
somesthetic sensation and, 82
Dorsiflexion, gait disorders and, 263
Double simultaneous stimulation, left-sided extinction to, 80
Double vision. *See* Diplopia
Dural sheaths, herniation and, 210
Dysarthria, 108
causes of, 138
functional classification of, 139
scanning, of cerebellar disease, 138
Dysconjugate gaze, 170–180
Dysmetria, and cerebellar lesions, 66

Ear, external, facial nerve pathway and, 254
Edema
and increased intracranial pressure, 156
after infarction, 194
Edinger-Westphal nuclei (EWN)
anisocoria and, 236
double vision and, 94
in pupillary light reflex pathway, 72
Efferent axons, and vocal cord paralysis, 64
Efferent pupillary defect versus afferent, in anisocoria, 232, 235, 236
Elbow, conduction block at, 224
Electromyography, lesion differentiation by, 238, 240
Embolus, amaurosis fugax and, 148
Endocarditis, 123
Ependymoma, 20, 269
Epidural hematoma, spinal cord lesion and, 20
Epilepsy, hemisphere involvement in, 194
Erb-Duchenne palsy, 241
Extensor hallucis longus muscle, 266
Extensor response, 204, 206

External genu, facial nerve pathway and, 254
Extinction, to double simultaneous stimulation, 80
Extraocular muscles, in eye movements, 206
Extrapyramidal disorders of gait, 262
Eye movements
  extraocular muscles in, 206
  oculovestibular, pathway for, 84
  pain and, 70
Eyelid
  and Bell's phenomenon, in unconsciousness, 198
  closure of, dysconjugate gaze and, 170
  ptosis of, 38
Eyes
  conjugate movement of, 32
  forced closure of, and Bell's phenomenon, 252
  misalignment of. See Diplopia
  right eye, vision loss in, 70

Facial anhidrosis
  in Horner's syndrome, 67
  sympathetic damage and, 236
Facial immobility. See Facial weakness
Facial muscles, facial nerve pathway and, 254
Facial nerve
  in abnormal corneal reflexes, 176
  and Bell's palsy, 256
  fasciculus, right-sided weakness and, 26
  nucleus
    corticobulbar fibers path to, 42
    innervation, 28
    pathway for, 82
    regions of, 28
    and supranuclear input from cerebral cortex, 254
  pathway of, facial weakness and, 254
Facial weakness, 252–256
  immobility, in left gaze paresis, 24
  left, and corticobulbar fiber lesion, 188
  motoneuron lesions and, 28, 140
  right, and left-sided weakness, 170, 174, 176
False localizing sign, brainstem lesion and, 210
Falx cerebri, 53
  herniation of, 210
  meningioma of, 54
Fasciculus
  arcuate. See Arcuate fasciculus
  facial nerve, 26
  medial longitudinal, 32
Femoral nerve, lower extremity muscles and, 265
Festination, 262

Finger-nose-finger test, in gait and truncal ataxia, 152
Finger-to-nose test
  in left-gaze paresis, 24
  in right-sided weakness, 38
Flaccid quadraparesis, coma and, 210
Flexor carpi ulnaris, weakness of, 220, 222–223
Flexor digiti minimi, weakness of, 220, 222–223
Flexor digitorum profundus, weakness of, 220, 222–223
Flocculonodular lobe
  injury to, 154
  vestibular system and, 154
Fluency
  Broca's area and, 144
  as parameter in aphasia, 110
Foramen magnum, herniation through, 210, 212
Foville's syndrome, 34
Frontal lobe, and optic chiasm compression, 96
Frontal transcallosal fibers, sympathetic apraxia and, 146
Frontopontine tract, 84
  lesion of, horizontal gaze and, 190

Gag reflex
  decreased consciousness and, 170
  in right palate paralysis, 64
Gait
  ataxia of, 152–156
  disorders of
    causes of, 262
    extrapyramidal, 262
    functional systems in, 262–263
    spastic, 262
  and upper motoneuron lesion, 26
Galactorrhea, and double vision, 92–96
Ganglion
  ciliary, in pupillary light reflex pathway, 72
  gasserian, in brainstem anatomy, 246
  geniculate, facial nerve pathway and, 254
  retinal, in pupillary light reflex pathway, 72
Gasserian ganglion, in brainstem anatomy, 246
Gastrocnemius muscle, wasting of, 260
Gaze
  conjugate
    systems in, 178
    volitional, 32
  dysconjugate, 170–180
  horizontal, control pathway for, 84, 85
  paresis, types of, 32
  supranuclear conjugate palsies of, 208

supranuclear disorder of, 84
voluntary
  control pathway for, 208
  loss of, 32
Geniculate ganglion, facial nerve pathway and, 254
Genu, external and internal, 254
Globe, and oculomotor nerve, 94
Glossopharyngeal nerve, hoarseness and, 64
Graphesthesia, 118, 120, 122
  medial lemniscus and, 82
Grave's disease, optic nerve lesion and, 74
Greater superficial petrosal nerve, facial weakness and, 254, 256
Guillain-Barré syndrome, 16
Gyrus, postcentral, somatesthetic sensation and, 82

Hallucinations, olfactory, 100–104
Hand, right, weakness and sensory loss in, 216–224
Head trauma, intracranial hematomas and, 54, 56
Headache
  and gait and truncal ataxia, 152–157
    pathologic possibilities for, 156
  increased intracranial pressure and, 194
  lower extremity weakness and, 48, 54
Heal-knee-shin test, in gait and truncal ataxia, 152
Hemangioma, optic nerve lesion and, 74
Hematoma
  epidural, 20
  and increased intracranial pressure, 156
  intracranial, head trauma and, 54, 56
  parasagittal subdural, 56
  subdural and epidural, unconsciousness and, 194
Hemianopsia. *See* Bitemporal hemianopsia; Homonymous hemianopsia
Hemiparesis, left, 206
Hemisphere disconnection syndromes, 132, 133. *See Also* Alexia
  apraxia and, 146
Hemispheres
  herniation in, 210, 212
  involvement in unresponsiveness, 206
Hemorrhage
  hypertensive
    intracerebral, 212
    unconsciousness and, 194
  and increased intracranial pressure, 156
  intracerebral, unconsciousness and, 194
  intracranial, unconsciousness and, 194
  intraparenchymal, 212

of spinal cord, 20
  left gaze paresis and, 34
  subarachnoid, 54
Herniation
  in hemispheres, 210
  syndromes of, 212
Hoarseness, 60, 62, 64
Hodgkin's disease
  right hand weakness in, 12
  spinal cord compression and, 20
Homonymous hemianopsia, 74, 75
  causes of, 128
  and retrochiasmal afferent visual system, 86
  and uncal herniation, 212
  and visual input, 130
Homonymous superior quadrantopsia, semicongruous right, 104
Hoover's sign, functional leg weakness and, 201
Horizontal diplopia, 42
  increased intracranial pressure and, 194
Horizontal gaze
  control pathway for, 84
  and tonic conjugate deviation of eyes, 190
Horizontal gaze palsy, 32
Horner's syndrome, 67
  dilatation lag in, 238
  and lateral pontine lesion, 180
  lesion differentiation in, 240
  miosis in, 67, 236
  sympathetic damage and, 236
Huntington's disease, chorea of, dysarthria and, 138
Hydrocephalus, and weakness of lower extremities, 54
Hydroxyamphetamine, and pupillary dilation, 240
Hyperacusis, facial weakness and, 254
Hyperreflexia
  unresponsiveness and ophthalmoplegia and, 204, 206
  and upper motoneuron lesion, 14
Hypertensive hemorrhage
  intracerebral, 212
  unconsciousness and, 194
Hypertonia, and left-sided weakness, 118, 120, 186
Hyperventilation, central neurogenic, coma and, 210
Hypotension, effect on watershed zone, 148
Hypothesis testing, in neurologic diagnosis, 4
Hypotonic deafferented bladder, 268

Idiopathic intracranial hypertension, 194
Illiteracy, versus alexia, 132
Immobility, facial. *See* Facial weakness

# Index

Infarction. *See* Vascular occlusion
Inferior cerebellar peduncle, in right-sided decreased sensation, 66
Inferior gluteal nerve, lower extremity muscles and, 265
Inferior oblique muscles
 in eye movements, 206
 innervation of, 44
Inferior recti muscles
 double vision and, 44
 in eye movements, 206
Inhibition, hyperreflexia and, 14
Intention tremor, 66
Intermediate region, of cerebellum, 154
 injury to, 154
Internal acoustic canal, facial nerve pathway and, 254
Internal capsule
 lesion of, in left arm ataxia and weakness, 164
 in voluntary gaze pathway, 208
Internal carotid artery
 in anterior circulation, 88
 in cavernous sinus, aneurysms of, 248
 emboli in, 148
 and optic chiasm compression, 96
Internal genu, facial nerve pathway and, 254
Intracerebral hemorrhage, unconsciousness and, 194
Intracranial cavity, volume determination of, 156
Intracranial hemorrhage, unconsciousness and, 194
Intracranial pressure, increase in
 abducens nerve palsies and, 208
 disorders causing, 194
 evidence for, 156
 methods for, 156
 papilledema and, 206
 unconsciousness and, 194
Intraparenchymal hemorrhages, 212
Ipsilateral cerebellum, lesions in, 66
Iris sphincter
 in pupillary light reflex pathway, 72
 innervation, anisocoria and, 235, 236
Ischemic optic neuropathy, 74

Labyrinth, stimulation of, in unconsciousness, 190
Lacrimal glands, facial weakness and, 254
Lacunar infarcts, common sites of, 166
Language system
 cortical regions involved in, 109, 110
 left hemisphere, apraxia and, 146
 lesions in. *See* Aphasia
 perisylvian language core in, 142
Lateral convexities, corticospinal fibers and, 52

Lateral funiculus, somatesthetic sensation and, 82
Lateral geniculate nucleus, in pupillary light reflex pathway, 72
Lateral medullary, lesion in, Horner's syndrome and, 67
Lateral nystagmus, quick phase in, unconsciousness and, 192
Lateral recti muscles, in eye movements, 206
Lateral zone, of cerebellum, 154
 injury to, 154
 left, limb ataxia and tremor and, 162
 lesion of efferent or afferent connections to, 164
 output origin of, 164
Left gaze paresis
 differential diagnosis in, 34
 left facial weakness and, 24
 left-sided weakness and, 80–89
 right-sided weakness and, 24–34
 visual field defect in, 80
Lemniscal system. *See* Medial lemniscus
Lesion
 for alexia, 130
 anatomic site identification, in neurologic diagnosis, 4, 6
 in atherosclerosis, site predilection for, 88
 of basis pontis, in left arm weakness, 164
 of brachium conjunctivum, in left arm weakness, 164
 in brain, and language difficulty, 109
 of brainstem, 30
 differential diagnosis of, 67
 in Brown-Séquard syndrome, 76
 cauda equina, walking difficulty and, 266
 in cerebellum, 66
 cortical, and right-sided weakness, 140
 of corticobulbar fibers
  left facial weakness and, 188
  left-sided weakness and, 206
  right-sided weakness and, 28
 of corticospinal tract
  left arm weakness and, 162, 164
  left-sided weakness and, 206
  right-sided weakness and, 14
 differentiation of
  by electromyography, 238, 240
  by pharmacologic testing, 240
 of dorsal columns, 154
 false localizing sign and, 210
 in gaze paresis, types causing, 32
 of internal capsule, in left arm weakness, 164
 in left pons, 30
 lower extremity weakness and, 50
 medullary, ataxic breathing and, 194

midline, medial convexities and, 52
in motor system, clinical findings for, 218, 219
in nucleus ambiguus, 64
of oculomotor nerve, 44
of parietal lobes, 122
pontine
  apneustic breathing and, 194
  in dysconjugate gaze, 176, 178
  in pupillary light reflex pathway, 72
  of retrochiasmal afferent visual system, 86
  of right C8–T1 nerve roots, in traumatic weakness, 238
right hemispinal cord, 18
in right-sided weakness
  in corticospinal tract, 14
  spinal compression and, 16
  in spinothalamic tract, 16
in right temporal lobe, 104
of spinothalamic tract
  right-sided weakness and, 16
  supratentorial, 210
of ulnar nerve, in right-handed weakness and sensory loss, 224
unilateral hemispheric, differential diagnosis in, 212
upper motoneuron, 26, 140
Lethargy, diencephalic dysfunction and, 210
Levator palpebrae muscle, innervation of, double vision and, 44
Long circumferential branches, anatomic localization of occulsion in, 166
Lower extremity weakness, 48–56
Lower motoneuron facial nerve nucleus, 28
Lower pontine–upper medulla stage breathing, in coma, 210
Lymphoma, Hodgkin's. *See* Hodgkin's disease

Malingering, unconsciousness and, 200
Marcus Gunn pupillary sign, 72
Maxillary division, of trigeminal nerve, facial numbness and, 244
Medial convexity, corticospinal fibers and, 52
Medial lemniscus
  balance impairment and, 154
  discriminative sensation mediation by, 16, 18
  dorsal root ganglion in, 18
  route of, 18
  and somatesthetic sensation, 82
Medial longitudinal fasciculus (MLF), 32
  and conjugate deviation of eyes, 192
  dysconjugate gaze and, 178
  horizontal gaze and, 190

Medial recti muscles
  double vision and, 44
  dysconjugate gaze and, 178
  in eye movements, 206
  horizontal gaze and, 190
Median nerve, conduction vulnerability site for, 224
Medulloblastoma, 156
Meningiomas, 20
  of cavernous sinus, facial numbness and, 248
  of falx cerebri, 54
Mesencephalic nucleus, facial anesthesia and, 62
Mesencephalon, oculomotor nucleus in, 94
Metacarpophalangeal joints, and claw hand deformity, 216
Metastasis, optic nerve lesion and, 74
Meyer's loop, 74
Micturition, processes in, 268
Middle cerebral artery, 88
  anatomic localization of occulsion in, 166
  and stroke symptoms, 88
Midline region, of cerebellum, 154
  injury to, 154
Miosis, in Horner's syndrome, 67, 236
Mixed transcortical aphasia, 133
MLF. *See* Medial longitudinal fasciculus (MLF)
Motoneuron. *See also* Anterior horn cell; Upper motoneuron
  alpha, reflexes and, 14
  from facial nerve, facial weakness and, 254
  in voluntary gaze pathway, 208
Motor cortex
  apraxia and, 146
  lesion of, 146
Motor function, of right upper extremity following trauma, 228
Motor nerve, peripheral, reflexes and, 14
Motor response, pathways of mediation for, 146
Motor systems, and speech difficulty. *See* Dysarthria
Müller's muscle, innervation of, Horner's syndrome and, 67, 236
Multiple sclerosis, 76
Muscle tone
  extraocular, 42
  measurement of, 14
  rectal, walking difficulty and, 260
  in right-sided weakness, 38, 40
Muscle wasting
  and anterior horn cell disease, 230
  causes of, 230
  following trauma to right arm, 228
  of legs, 260

Muscle wasting—*Continued*
  segmental innervation, in lower extremity, 264, 265
Muscles
  abductor digiti minimi, weakness of, 220, 222–223
  abductor pollicis, weakness of, 220, 222–223
  bulbocavernous reflex, walking difficulty and, 260
  detrusor, bladder dysfunction and, 268
  disease of, gait disorders and, 262
  dorsal interossei, weakness of, 220, 222–223
  extensor hallucis longus, walking difficulty and, 266
  facial, weakness of, 252–256
  flexor carpi ulnaris, weakness of, 220, 222–223
  flexor digiti minimi, weakness of, 220, 222–223
  flexor digitorum profundus, weakness of, 220, 222–223
  gastrocnemius, 260
  inferior oblique
    in eye movements, 206
    innervation of, 44
  inferior recti
    in double vision, 44
    in eye movements, 206
  innervation of
    in double vision, 44
    Müller's, 67, 236
    by peripheral nerves, 232, 234–235
    segmental, of lower limbs, 264, 265
  lateral recti, in eye movements, 206
  lesion of, clinical findings for, 218, 219
  levator palpebrae, double vision and, 44
  lower extremity strength of, 260
  medial recti. *See* Medial recti muscles
  opponens digiti minimi, weakness of, 220, 222–223
  palmar interossei, weakness of, 220, 222–223
  peripheral, myopathy and, 218
  and right upper extremity motor functions, 228
  soleus, 260
  stapedius, facial nerve pathway and, 254
  superior oblique
    in eye movements, 206
    innervation of, 44
    trochlear nerve and, 44
  superior recti
    in double vision, 44
    in eye movements, 206
  tibialis anterior, walking difficulty and, 266
  tone of. *See* Muscle tone
  of upper extremity
    innervation of, 232, 234–235
    table of, 222–223
  wasting of. *See* Muscle wasting
Myopathy
  gait disorders and, 262
  peripheral muscle weakness and, 218

Nasolabial fold, loss in right facial weakness, 176
Nausea
  increased intracranial pressure and, 194
  vestibular dysfunction and, 66
Nerve conduction studies, right-handed weakness and sensory loss and, 224
Nerve roots
  C8–T1. *See* C8–T1 nerve roots
  and innervation of upper extremity muscles, 232, 234–235
  in lower spine, walking difficulty and, 266
  sacral, sexual dysfunction and, 268
  sympathetic ganglia and chain relationship to, 238
  traumatic damage to, 230
Nerves
  abducens. *See* Abducens nerve
  auditory, facial nerve pathway and, 254
  common peroneal, conduction vulnerability site for, 224
  cranial
    in brainstem anatomy, 246, 247
    double vision and, 92
  facial. *See* Facial nerve
  femoral, lower extremity muscles and, 265
  glossopharyngeal, hoarseness and, 64
  greater superficial petrosal, facial weakness and, 254, 256
  inferior gluteal, lower extremity muscles and, 265
  intermediate, somatesthetic sensation and, 254
  median, conduction vulnerability site for, 224
  obdurator, lower extremity muscles and, 265
  oculomotor. *See* Oculomotor nerve
  olfactory
    factitious anosmia and, 200
    in olfactory system anatomy, 102
  optic, in pupillary light reflex pathway, 72, 74, 75
  peripheral. *See* Peripheral nerves

radial, conduction vulnerability site
  for, 224
 roots of. See C8–T1 nerve roots; Nerve
  roots
 sciatic, lower extremity muscles and,
  265
 spinal, anatomy of, 238
 spinal cord, exit of, 220
 superior gluteal, lower extremity muscles and, 265
 trigeminal. See Trigeminal nerve
 trochlear. See Trochlear nerve
 ulnar, sensory loss and weakness of
  right hand and, 224
 vagus
  route of, 65
  and vocal cord innervation, 64
 vestibulocochlear
  clumsiness and, 66
  and conjugate deviation of eyes, 192
Neural foramina, in neural anatomy, 220
Neurofibromas, 20
Neuromuscular junction, 14
 lesion of, clinical findings for, 218, 219
Noxious stimulation
 in unconsciousness, 174, 184, 186, 188,
  198, 200
 unresponsiveness and, 204
Nucleus ambiguus, and vocal cord paralysis, 64
Nucleus solitarius, facial weakness and,
 254
Numbness
 facial, and double vision, 244–248
 of left arm and leg, 12–20
 left-sided, 70–76
 of right arm, with anisocoria, 228–241
Nystagmus
 horizontal, lateral gaze and, 60
 lateral, caloric testing and, 190
 left-beating horizontal, following ice
  water irrigation, 198
 vestibular dysfunction and, 66

Obdurator nerve, lower extremity muscles and, 265
Obicularis oris, facial weakness and, 30
Oblique muscles, eye movements and,
 206
Obstructive hydrocephalus, increased intracranial pressure and, 194
Occipital lobe, lesion characteristics of,
 104
Occlusion. See Vascular occlusion
Ocular sympathetic pathways, anisocoria
 and, 236
Oculocephalic maneuver. See Doll's-head
 maneuver

Oculomotor nerve
 and brachium conjunctivum lesion,
  164
 in brainstem anatomy, 246
 and conjugate deviation of eyes,
  192
 in double vision, 44
 in eye movements, 206
 functions of, 94
 innervation by, 44
 in left gaze paresis, 32
 nucleus of, 94
 in pupillary light reflex pathway, 72
Oculomotor nerve palsy, and uncal herniation, 212
Oculovestibular eye movements, pathway for, 84
Olfactory bulb, in olfactory system anatomy, 102
Olfactory hallucinations, 100–104
Olfactory nerve, factitious anosmia and,
 200
Olfactory sensory epithelium, seizure
 discharge in, 102
Olfactory system anatomy, 102
 olfactory tubercle, 102
 olfactory nerve in, 102
Oligodendroglioma, 104
ON. See Optic nerve
Ophthalmic artery, left visual field loss
 and, 88
Ophthalmic artery, platelet-thrombin
 embolus in, 148
Ophthalmic division, of trigeminal nerve,
 facial numbness and, 244
Ophthalmoplegia, unresponsiveness and,
 204–212
Opponens digiti minimi, weakness of,
 220, 222–223
Optic chiasm
 double vision and, 96
 lesions of, 74, 75
 and pituitary gland relationship, 96
 in pupillary light reflex pathway, 72
 and right visual field loss, 128
Optic nerve
 glioma of, 74
 in pupillary light reflex pathway, 72
 right, lesion in, 72, 74, 75
Optic nerve sheath meningioma, 74
Optic neuritis, 74
Optic radiations, right-sided lesions and,
 86
Optic tract
 lesion characteristics of, 104
 in pupillary light reflex pathway, 72
Orbital frontal cortex, partial complex
 seizures of, 102

281

# Index

Pain
- spinal trigeminal nucleus and, 62
- and spinothalamic pathway lesions, 188

Palmar interossei, weakness of, 220, 222–223

Palsy
- of abducens nerve, 210
- Bell's, 256
- Dejerine-Klumpke, 241
- Erb-Duchenne, 241
- horizontal gaze, 32
- oculomotor nerve, in uncal herniation, 212
- Saturday night, 224

Papilledema
- increased intracranial pressure and, 54, 194, 206
- lower extremity weakness and, 48
- ophthalmoplegia and, 204

Paralysis
- facial. See Facial weakness
- of right palate, 64
- of vocal cords, 64

Paramedian pontine reticular formation (PPRF)
- and abducens nuclear complex, ice-water stimulation of, 192
- dysconjugate gaze and, 178
- facial nucleus and, 254
- frontopontine tract and, 84
- horizontal gaze and, 190
- right-sided weakness and, 32
- voluntary gaze and, 208

Paraphasia, 108

Parasagittal subdural hematoma, 56

Parasympathetic pathways, anisocoria and, 236

Parasympathetic stimulation, of pupils, 236

Paravermal region, of cerebellum, 154
- injury to, 154

Paresis
- of abducens nerve, 194
- left gaze. See Left gaze paresis

Parietal lobe
- abscess of, 123
- lesion characteristics of, 104
- and perceptual disturbances, 122

Parkinson's disease
- dysarthria and, 128
- gait disorders and, 262

Patellar tendon reflex, 60

Pattern recognition, in neurologic diagnosis, 4

Perception
- disturbances of, 118–123
- picture recognition and, 118
- pinprick, and spinothalamic tracts, 16, 120

Perimetry visual field testing, in double vision, 92

Peripheral nerves
- and innervation of upper extremity muscles, 232, 234–235
- lesion of, clinical findings for, 218, 219
- of muscles of upper extremity, 223
- reflexes and, 14
- sectioning, in traumatic weakness, 230
- of upper extremities, 220

Peripheral vision, in right eye, 70

Perisylvian language core, anomia and, 142

Pharmacologic testing, and lesion differentiation, in Horner's syndrome, 240

Pinprick sensation, spinalthalamic system and, 16, 120

Pituitary adenoma, prolactin secretion from, 96

Pituitary gland, and optic chiasm relationship, 96

Plexus
- brachial. See Brachial plexus
- venous, in cavernous sinus, 248

Pons
- left
  - infarct of, 34
  - lesion in, 30
- lower
  - and left-sided weakness, 174
  - and motor system lesion, 82

Postcentral gyrus, somatesthetic sensation and, 82

Posterior cerebral artery
- anatomic localization of occlusion in, 166
- and uncal herniation, 212
- and visual loss, 88

Posterior circulation
- in brain arterial system, 88
- disease signs and symptoms in, 88

Posterior communicating artery, 88

Posterior inferior cerebellar artery
- anatomic localization of occlusion in, 166
- in posterior circulation, 88

Posterior ramus, spinal nerve and, 238

Posterior spinal artery, anatomic localization of occlusion in, 166

PPRF. See Paramedian pontine reticular formation (PPRF)

Premotor cortex, lesion of, 146

Pretectal nucleus, (PTN), in pupillary light reflex pathway, 72

Principal sensory nucleus, facial anesthesia and, 62

Prolactinoma, 96

Proprioception
- and left-sided weakness, 80

medial lemniscal system and, 16, 18
and mesancephalic nucleus, 62
Pseudotumor cerebri, increased intracranial pressure and, 194
Ptosis, 38
  differential diagnosis in, 44
  left, and facial numbness, 244
  and oculomotor nerve lesion, 44
  partial, in Horner's syndrome, 67
  pathological findings in, 44
  sympathetic damage and, 236
  traumatic weakness and, 232
Pupillary defects, afferent versus efferent, in anisocoria, 232, 235, 236
Pupillary light reflex, 70
  anisocoria and, 236
  in double vision, 92
  pathway for, 72
Pupillomiosis, 236
Pupils. *See also* Pupillary light reflex
  afferent versus efferent defects, in anisocoria, 232, 235, 236
  coma and, 210
  constriction of, 72
  dilation of, pharmacologic agents for, 240
  in double vision, 92
  light reactivity of, 24
    in right-sided weakness, 38
  miosis of, in Horner's syndrome, 67
Pure alexia. *See* Alexia
Pure word deafness, 133
Putamen, lesions in, and language disturbance, 109
Pyramidal system. *See* Corticospinal tract
Pyriform lobe, in olfactory system anatomy, 102

Quadrantopsia, semicongruous right homonymous superior, 104
Quadraparesis, flaccid, coma and, 210
Quick phase, in lateral nystagmus, 192

Radial nerve, conduction vulnerability site for, 224
Ramus, spinal nerve and, 238
Rathke's pouch, and bitemporal hemianopsias, 96
Reactive automatisms, 102
Reading
  alexia and, 126–133
  disorders of, 133
Rectal tone, walking difficulty and, 260
Rectus muscles
  eye movements and, 206
  oculomotor nerve innervation of, 44
Reflex
  bulbocavernous, walking difficulty and, 260
  corneal, and trigeminal nerve mediation, 62
  patellar tendon, 60
  pupillary light. *See* Pupillary light reflex
  requirements for, 14
Respiration
  apneustic, 194
  ataxic, 194
  unconscious, left-sided weakness and, 184–194
Respiratory patterns, factors affecting, 194
Retina
  image position disparity in, 42
  inferior and superior, in afferent visual system anatomy, 104
Retinal artery, platelet-thrombin embolus in, 148
Retinal ganglion cell (RET), in pupillary light reflex pathway, 72
Right hemispinal cord lesion, 18
Romberg's sign
  absence of, 60
  balance impairment and, 154
  elicitation of, 66
  and factitious ataxia, 201
Roots, of muscles of upper extremity, 222
Ruptured aneurysms, unconsciousness and, 194

Sacral cord, bladder dysfunction and, 268
Salivary glands, facial weakness and, 254
Saturday night palsy, 224
Scanning dysarthria, 138
Schwannomas, 20
Sciatic nerve, lower extremity muscles and
  peroneal nerve and, 265
  tibial nerve and, 265
Seizure
  generalized tonic clonic, 118
  and olfactory hallucinations, 102
  partial complex, symptoms in, 102
  positive symptoms in, 100
  symptoms associated with, 86
Sella turcica, and optic chiasm compression, 96
Sensation. *See also* Perception
  absence with right-sided weakness, 16
  cortical, 122
  decrease in right side, 60–67
  discriminative, and parietal damage, 122
  and lower extremity weakness, 48
  and midline lesion in cerebral cortex, 52
  primary and cortical modalities of, 82

# Index

Sensation—*Continued*
somatesthetic
facial weakness and, 254
left-sided weakness and, 82
Sensory loss, 60–67
and damage to parietal regions, 122
and weakness in right hand, 216–224
Sensory modalities, primary and cortical, 82
Septal nuclei, in olfactory system anatomy, 102
Short circumferential branches, anatomic localization of occlusion of, 166
Sinus
cavernous. *See* Cavernous sinus
superior sagittal, head trauma and, 56
Skull
content composition of, 156
trauma to, 56
Slurring, of speech, 24
and left pons lesion, 30
Small end arteries, occlusion of, and left arm weakness, 166
Smile, symmetry in facial weakness, 28
Soft palate, paralysis of, 64
Soleus muscle, wasting of, 260
Somatesthetic sensation
facial weakness and, 254
left-sided weakness and, 82
Somatosensory cortex, 82
Somesthetic sensation. *See* Somatesthetic sensation
Spastic bladder, 268
Spastic gait, 262
Speech. *See also* Aphasia; Dysarthria
comprehension of. *See* Auditory comprehension
difficulty, and right-sided weakness, 136–148
fluency of. *See* Fluency
hoarseness of, 60, 62, 64
slurring of, 24
and left pons lesion, 30
sudden difficulty in, 108–115
Sphincter function, bladder dysfunction and, 268
Spinal cord
cervical, right-sided weakness and, 14
compression of, 16
Hodgkin's lymphoma and, 20
corticospinal fibers in, 52
and corticospinal tract lesion, 82, 83
hemorrhage of, 20
lesions of dorsal column, balance and, 154
nerves exit from, 220
relationship with zones of cerebellum, 154

right-side lesions, Brown-Séquard syndrome and, 76
traumatic nerve damage to roots in, 230
and vertebral column development, 266
Spinal nerve, anatomy of, 238
Spinal trigeminal nucleus, function of, 62
Spinothalamic tract
and Brown-Séquard syndrome, 76
contralateral trigeminal system and, lesion in, 62
left-sided weakness and, 180
and pain mediation, 188
and perceptual disturbances, 120
route of, 16
and somatesthetic sensation, 82
Stapedius muscle, facial nerve pathway and, 254
Stereognosis, 122
Stereotyped automatisms, 102
Stimulation
and nervous system levels, 6
noxious
in unconsciousness, 174, 184, 186, 188, 198, 200
unresponsiveness and, 204
of pupils, parasympathetic versus sympathetic, 236
Stroke
and anterior cerebral artery, 88
causes of, 114, 115
versus tumors, 34
Subarachnoid hemorrhage, 54
Submaxillary gland, facial nerve pathway and, 254
Superior bilateral quadrantanopsia, 94
Superior cerebral artery, anatomic localization of occlusion in, 166
Superior gluteal nerve, lower extremity muscles and, 265
Superior oblique muscles
in eye movements, 206
trochlear nerve and, 44
Superior recti muscles
double vision and, 44
in eye movements, 206
Superior sagittal sinus, head trauma and, 56
Superior salivary nucleus, facial weakness and, 254
Supranuclear disorder of gaze, 84
Supranuclear fibers, facial weakness and, 254
"Swinging flashlight test," pupillary light reflex and, 72
Sylvian fissure, language system and, 109
Sympathetic apraxia, 133
and lesion of Broca's area, 146

Sympathetic pathways, ocular, anisocoria and, 236
Sympathetic stimulation, of pupils, 236

Tabes dorsalis, gait disorders and, 263
Tactile information, principal sensory nucleus and, 62
Tarsal muscle of Müller, 67
Taste, loss of, facial weakness and, 254, 256
Tearing, facial weakness and, 254, 256
Temperature
  spinal trigeminal nucleus and, 62
  spinalthalamic system and, 16
Temporal lobe
  olfactory system and, 102
  and optic chiasm compression, 96
  partial complex seizures of, 102
  right, lesion in, 104
  and speech perception, 110
  and uncal herniation, 212
Tendon reflexes, and right-sided weakness, 136
Tentorium cerebelli, herniation of, 210
Tentorium notch
  in central transtentorial herniation, 210
  uncal herniation and, 212
Thalamus
  lesions in, and language disturbance, 109
  somatesthetic sensation and, 82
Tibialis anterior muscle, walking difficulty and, 266
Tone, of muscles. *See* Muscle tone
Tongue, facial nerve pathway and, 254, 255
Transient visual loss. *See* Amaurosis fugax
Trauma
  to head, 54, 56
  right arm weakness from, 228–241
Tremor
  ataxia and, 162
  intention, 66
Trigeminal nerve
  in abnormal corneal reflexes, 176
  in brainstem anatomy, 246
  divisions of, facial numbness and, 244
  factitious anosmia and, 200
  functions of, 62
Trochlear nerve
  in brainstem anatomy, 246
  in eye movements, 206
  functions of, 94
  superior oblique muscle and, 44
  in voluntary gaze pathway, 208
Truncal ataxia, 152–156

Tumor
  alexia and, 130
  of cavernous sinus, facial numbness and, 248
  and increase in brain compartment, 156
  of left cerebral peduncle, 44
  metastatic, 20
  versus strokes, 34
Two-point discrimination, left-sided weakness and, 122

Ulnar nerve, sensory loss and weakness of right hand and, 224
Uncal herniation, 212
Unconsciousness. *See also* Consciousness
  left-sided weakness and
    altered respirations in, 184–194
    dysconjugate gaze in, 170–180
  with normal findings, 198–201
  psychiatric evaluation in, 201
  spontaneous recovery from, 201
Unresponsiveness, and ophthalmoplegia, 204–212
Upper medulla, and nucleus ambiguus lesion, 64
Upper motoneuron
  facial nerve nucleus, 26, 28
  lesion of, clinical findings for, 218, 219
  lesion, and right facial weakness, 140
  right-sided weakness and, 26
Upward transtentorial herniation, 212
Urinary bladder dysfunction, 260–269

Vagus nerve, and vocal cord innervation, 64
Vascular occlusion, 20
  aphasia and, 114
  in brain parenchyma, 115
  in left anterior cerebral arterial distribution, 148
  left gaze paresis and, 34
  left-sided weakness and, 86, 180
  at watershed zone border, 148
Venous plexus, in cavernous sinus, 248
Ventral trigeminal tract, 62
Verbal command, and motor response pathways, 146
Vermal region, of cerebellum, 154
  injury to, 154
Vertebral artery
  in posterior circulation, 88
  thrombosis of, 67
Vertebral column, and spinal cord development, 266
Vertigo, vestibular dysfunction and, 66
Vestibular system
  clumsiness and, 66

# Index

Vestibular system—*Continued*
  and conjugate deviation of eyes, 192
  and midline zone of cerebellum, 154
Vestibulocochlear nerve
  clumsiness and, 66
  and conjugate deviation of eyes, 192
Vestibuloocular pathway, ophthalmoplegia and, 208
Vestibuloocular reflex, coma and, 210
Vibration
  conversion reaction and, 200
  medial lemniscal system and, 16, 18, 19
Visual acuity, 70
  and right visual field loss, 126
Visual confrontation naming, in aphasia, 108
Visual field
  defect in left gaze paresis, 80
  in double vision
    confrontational testing and, 92
    perimetry testing and, 92
  inferior and superior, in afferent visual system anatomy, 104
  left, loss of, 80–88
  and lesions of optic chiasm, 74, 75
  olfactory hallucinations and, 100
  right, loss of, 126–133
  temporal, and nasal retina, 96
  and visual loss in right eye, 70
Visual loss
  with olfactory hallucinations, 100–104
  in right eye, 70–76
  transient. *See* Amaurosis fugax
Visual system, afferent, pathway subserving, 74, 75
Visual threshold, 70
Vocal cord
  innervation of, 64
  paralysis, 64
Voluntary gaze
  control pathway for, 208
  loss of, 32

Vomiting, increased intracranial pressure and, 194

Walking, difficulty. *See also* Gait, disorders of
  and urinary bladder dysfunction, 260–269
Wallenberg's syndrome, 67
Wasting, of muscles. *See* Muscles wasting
Watershed zone, effect of hypotension on, 148
Weakness
  asymmetry, in lower extremities, 260
  of both lower extremities, 48–56
  facial. *See* Facial weakness
  of left arm, 160–166
  left-sided, 80–88
    dysconjugate gaze and, 170–180
    ophthalmoplegia and, 204, 206
    and perceptual disturbances, 118–123
    respiratory change and, 184–194
  proximal, gait disorders and, 262
  of right arm and leg, 12–20
  right-sided
    and double vision, 38–44
    and left gaze paresis, 24–34
    and speech difficulty, 136–148
    and visual loss, 70–76
  and sensory loss in right hand, 216–224
  traumatic, of right arm, 228–241
Weber's syndrome, 44
Wernicke's area
  anatomy of, 109
  and auditory comprehension, 112
  function of, 110
  and posterior left hemisphere occlusion, 148
  verbal comprehension and, 144
Word-finding difficulty. *See* Anomia